CLINICAL PORTFOLIO

Clinical and Employability Skills for Health Care Professions

Debra Borchert

Linda Stanhope

Kimberly Turnbull

Publisher
The Goodheart-Willcox Company, Inc.
Tinley Park, IL
www.g-w.com

ISBN 979-8-89448-602-4

1 2 3 4 5 6 7 8 9 – 26 – 29 28 27 26 25 24

Front Cover Image Credits: SDI Productions/iStock/Getty Images Plus via Getty Images; Ivan Pantic/iStock/Getty Images Plus via Getty Images; Wavebreakmedia/iStock/Getty Images Plus via Getty Images

Guided Tour

The instructional design includes student-focused learning tools to help students succeed. This visual guide highlights the features designed for the digital program through G-W Ignite.

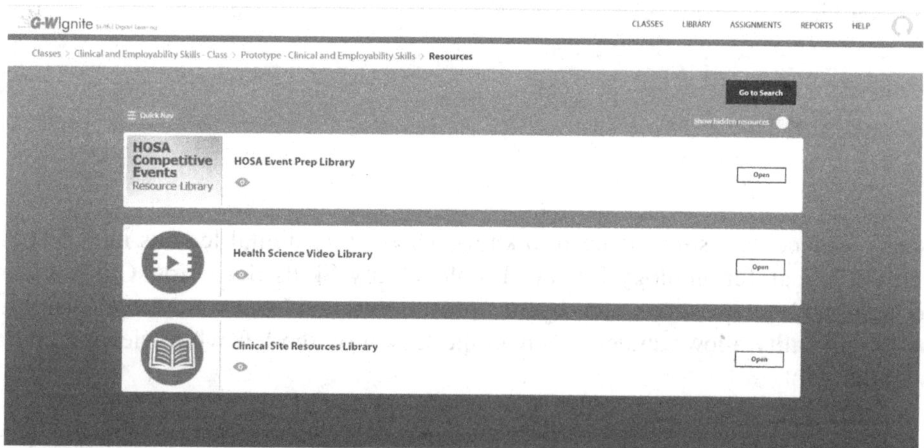

HOSA Event Prep Library includes practice activities for specific HOSA events, aligned to the appropriate student lesson(s).

Health Science Video Library includes videos and quizzes designed to support your health science education, aligned to the appropriate student lesson(s).

Clinical Resources Library includes additional resources for instructors to ensure your students are prepared for each clinical experience.

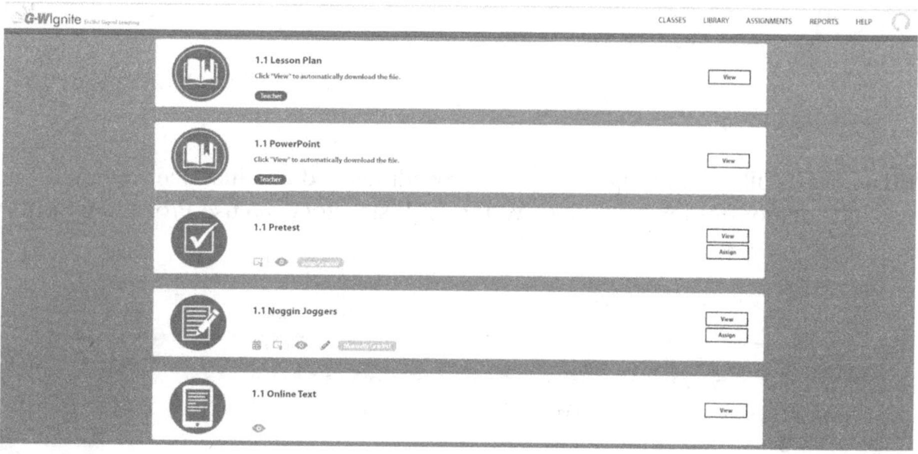

Learning Path organization within G-W Ignite keeps all resources for each lesson in one, easy-to-access location. View, assign, and customize your resources in the order that best meets your needs.

Lesson Plans guide you through content day by day.

PowerPoint® Presentations contain all student lesson content and are customizable to meet your needs.

Pretests, Posttests, and Exams assess student understanding of material.

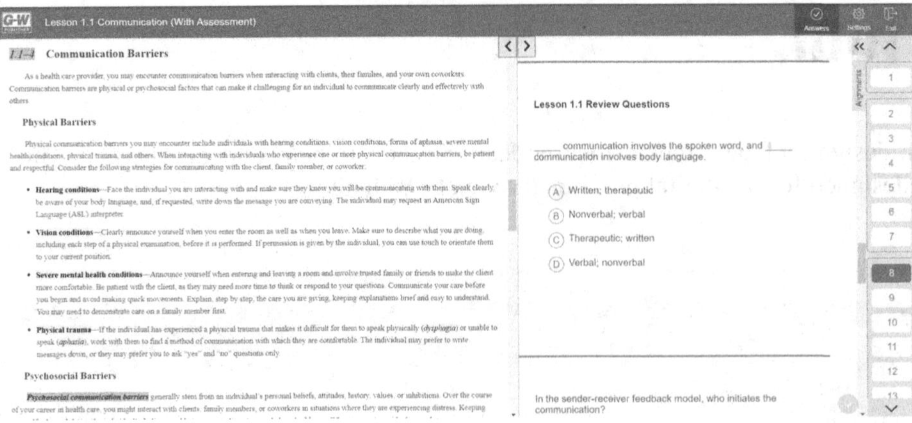

Student Lessons cover content students need to know. These fully digital lessons include Learning Outcomes, Key Terms, a Medical Terminology Review, Employability Skills Scenarios, Clinical Case Studies, Think About It critical thinking questions, step-by-step procedures, and Lesson Review questions.

Reading Pane functionality allows students to read the lesson on the left while viewing and answering review questions on the right.

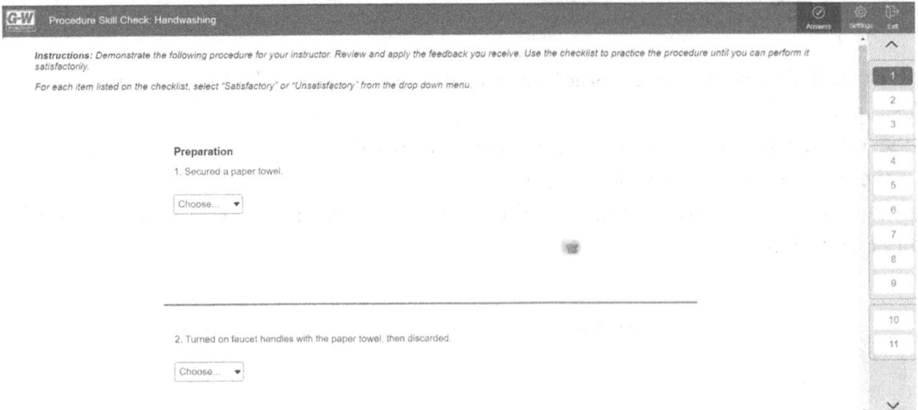

Procedure Skills Checks allow students to practice procedures and conduct peer review, either in person or by uploading a video demonstration through G-W Ignite. Instructors can use Procedure Skills Checks as assessment tools.

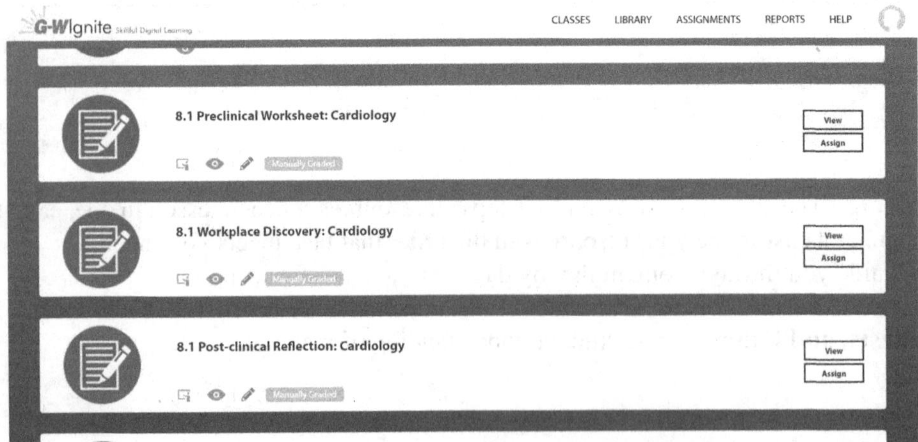

Clinical Portfolio contains Pre-Clinical Worksheets, Workplace Discovery Sheets, and Post-Clinical Reflections that students can utilize before, during, and after each clinical experience.

Contents

Radiology Services

Rehabilitation

Reproductive Health

Skeletomuscular

Surgery

Urinary

Name ______________________ Date ____________ Period ____________

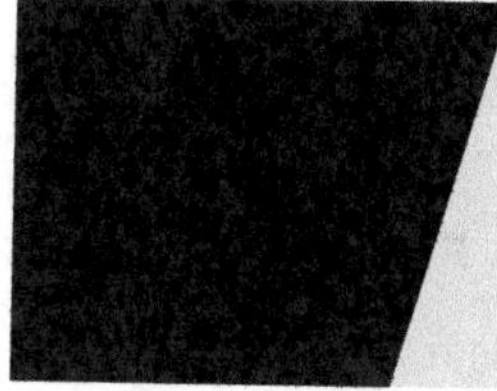

Biomedical Equipment Pre-Clinical Worksheet

Instructions: Answer the following questions.

1. What type of education is required to be a biomedical equipment technician?

2. Research the difference between a biomedical engineer and a biomedical equipment technician.

   A. Education requirements

   Biomedical engineer:

   Biomedical equipment technician:

   B. Job description

   Biomedical engineer:

   Biomedical equipment technician:

   C. Salary

   Biomedical engineer:

   Biomedical equipment technician:

   D. Workplace setting

   Biomedical engineer:

   Biomedical equipment technician:

(Continued)

E. Job outlook

Biomedical engineer:

Biomedical equipment technician:

3. List three types of equipment that a biomedical equipment technician works with often. Then, explain what the equipment is used for.

A. Equipment #1

Type:

Use:

B. Equipment #2

Type:

Use:

C. Equipment #3

Type:

Use:

Name ______________________ Date ____________ Period ____________

Biomedical Equipment Workplace Discovery Sheet

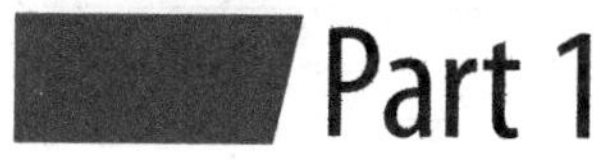

Part 1

During the Clinical Experience

Instructions: Answer the following questions.

1. What does a biomedical equipment technician do?

2. What education and training are necessary to work as a biomedical equipment technician?

3. What equipment do you enjoy working with the most? Least?

4. Do you have to go through other training when the hospital buys new equipment?

5. Is your team responsible for training the hospital staff to run new equipment?

6. What type of equipment requires daily maintenance by your department? Or is daily maintenance done by the staff who works with that equipment?

7. What type of equipment requires weekly maintenance? Monthly?

8. What do you like most about this career?

(Continued)

9. What advice would you have for others who want to do similar work?

____

____

10. What additional courses do you wish you had taken in high school or college?

____

____

11. In a typical work week, how much of your time do you spend fixing equipment?

____

____

12. What is quality assurance?

____

____

13. What medical terms or abbreviations do you commonly use?

____

____

Part 2

After the Clinical Experience

Instructions: For each item below, identify whether you observed or assisted. Then, provide a brief summary.

Orientation

1. Equipment assessment/analyzers
   ☐ Observed
   ☐ Assisted
   Brief summary:

   ____

   ____

2. Emergency procedures
   ☐ Observed
   ☐ Assisted
   Brief summary:

   ____

   ____

(Continued)

Name ____

Equipment

3. X-ray machines
   ☐ Observed
   ☐ Assisted
   Brief summary:
   ____
   ____

4. IV infusion pumps
   ☐ Observed
   ☐ Assisted
   Brief summary:
   ____
   ____

5. Telemetry monitors
   ☐ Observed
   ☐ Assisted
   Brief summary:
   ____
   ____

6. Electronic thermometers
   ☐ Observed
   ☐ Assisted
   Brief summary:
   ____
   ____

7. Pulse oximeters
   ☐ Observed
   ☐ Assisted
   Brief summary:
   ____
   ____

8. Ventilators/respirators
   ☐ Observed
   ☐ Assisted
   Brief summary:
   ____
   ____

(Continued)

9. CT scans

☐ Observed

☐ Assisted

Brief summary:

____

____

10. MRI

☐ Observed

☐ Assisted

Brief summary:

____

____

11. Ultrasound

☐ Observed

☐ Assisted

Brief summary:

____

____

12. Echocardiograph

☐ Observed

☐ Assisted

Brief summary:

____

____

13. Dopplers

☐ Observed

☐ Assisted

Brief summary:

____

____

14. Fetal monitors

☐ Observed

☐ Assisted

Brief summary:

____

____

(Continued)

Name ___________________________________

15. Electrocardiograph
    ☐ Observed
    ☐ Assisted
    Brief summary:
    ____
    ____

16. Holter monitors
    ☐ Observed
    ☐ Assisted
    Brief summary:
    ____
    ____

17. Defibrillators
    ☐ Observed
    ☐ Assisted
    Brief summary:
    ____
    ____

18. Lasers
    ☐ Observed
    ☐ Assisted
    Brief summary:
    ____
    ____

19. Telecommunication equipment
    ☐ Observed
    ☐ Assisted
    Brief summary:
    ____
    ____

20. Computers
    ☐ Observed
    ☐ Assisted
    Brief summary:
    ____
    ____

(Continued)

21. Electroencephalograph
    ☐ Observed
    ☐ Assisted
    Brief summary:

    ____

    ____

Other

22. Routine maintenance
    ☐ Observed
    ☐ Assisted
    Brief summary:

    ____

    ____

23. Quality assurance
    ☐ Observed
    ☐ Assisted
    Brief summary:

    ____

    ____

Student Name: ______________________________

Technician Name: ______________________________

Student ______________________ Dates ____________ Site ____________ Preceptor ____________

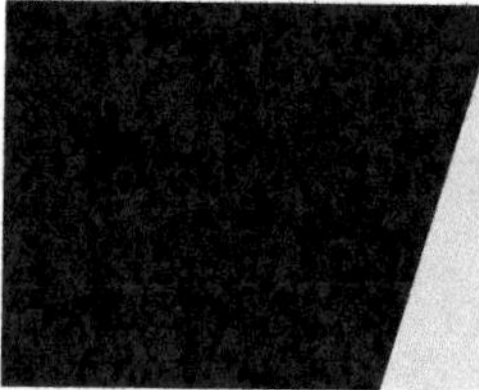

Biomedical Equipment Post-Clinical Reflection

Rotation Report

Overview

Instructions: Answer the following questions using complete sentences.

1. What were your responsibilities or duties this week?

____

____

2. What new knowledge or skill did you learn or observe this week?

____

____

3. What was the best thing that happened at your clinical site this week?

____

____

4. What was the most challenging thing that happened at your clinical site this week?

____

____

5. What problems or difficulties did you encounter or observe at your clinical site? How were they dealt with?

____

____

6. Was this week good, fair, or bad? Explain.

____

____

Observations

Instructions: List the observations you made for each of the following categories.

1. Technology observed:

____

____

2. Diagnostic procedures observed:

____

____

(Continued)

3. Therapeutic procedures observed:

____

____

4. Diseases or disorders observed:

____

____

5. Medical terminology or abbreviations encountered:

____

____

6. Other observations:

____

____

Supervisor Signature: ______________________________

Date: ______________________________

Rotation Journal

Instructions: Write a journal entry detailing your learning experience at the clinical rotation. Use the following topics to help write a complete journal entry.

Assessment of the Environment

- Personnel
- Services provided
- Equipment
- Technology utilized

Observation

- Health care providers
- Team skills
- Communication skills
- Safety procedures
- Therapeutic/diagnostic procedures

Knowledge

- New information learned
- Medical terminology
- Skills learned

Evaluation

- Personal experience
- Educational value
- Professional value

Journal Entry

Write a journal entry summarizing your clinical experience.

____

____

____

____

____

____

Name ______ Date ______ Period ______

Cardiopulmonary Pre-Clinical Worksheet

Instructions: Answer the following questions.

1. Label the parts of the heart.

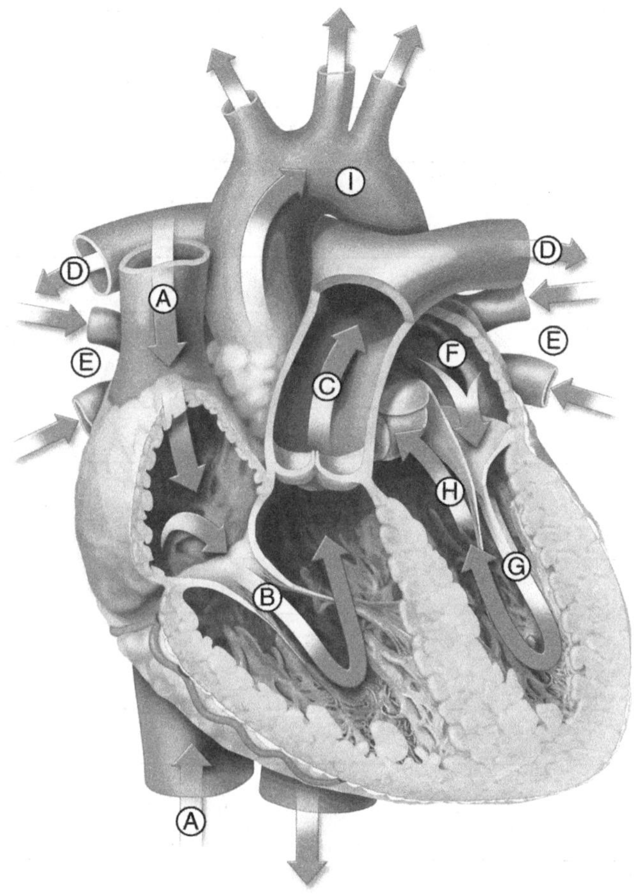

© Body Scientific International

A. ______

B. ______

C. ______

D. ______

E. ______

F. ______

G. ______

H. ______

I. ______

(Continued)

2. What diagnostic tests can be done to evaluate heart function?

3. Define the following terms:

A. Angina:

B. Arrhythmia:

C. Asystole:

D. Cardiomyopathy:

E. Cardioversion:

F. Depolarization:

G. Echocardiography:

H. Ectopic beat:

I. Fibrillation:

J. Ischemia:

K. Myocardial infarction:

(Continued)

Name ___

L. Sinus arrhythmia:

M. Thrombosis:

4. What is an EKG/ECG?

5. Explain where EKG leads are placed and why.

6. Examine the following EKG strips and explain how the different patterns affect heart function.

A. Normal sinus rhythm

B. Sinus bradycardia

C. Sinus tachycardia

PACs

D. Sinus rhythm with PACs

E. Atrial fibrillation

PVCs

F. Every other beat is a PVC

G. Ventricular tachycardia

H. Ventricular fibrillation

I. Third-degree heart block

7. How can a myocardial infarction be identified on an EKG strip?

8. Explain why EKGs are performed during stress testing and what changes occur to the EKG when there is heart damage.

9. What does asystole look like on an EKG?

(Continued)

10. Identify the risk factors for cardiovascular disease.

11. Compare and contrast angioplasty, atherectomy, and bypass surgery.

12. What are the signs and symptoms of a cerebrovascular accident (CVA)?

13. Differentiate between atherosclerosis and arteriosclerosis.

14. What are the signs and symptoms of a heart attack?

15. What is a Holter monitor, and when is one indicated?

16. Differentiate between bradycardia and tachycardia.

17. Explain the difference between systolic and diastolic pressure.

18. What are normal systolic and diastolic pressures for an adult?

19. What are normal pulse rates for an adult?

20. What would you expect for a normal pulse rate of a triathlete?

Name ________________ Date ________ Period ________

Cardiopulmonary Workplace Discovery Sheet

Part 1

During the Clinical Experience

Instructions: Answer the following questions.

1. What does a cardiologist do?

2. To work on the cath lab team requires experts from different backgrounds medically. What are the different backgrounds for your team?

3. What education and training are necessary to work as a telemetry nurse?

4. What is the average number of clients seen on a daily basis in the cath lab?

5. What is the educational background needed to perform echocardiograms?

6. Who interprets the results of an echocardiogram?

7. How many EKGs are typically performed each day?

8. Who reads and interprets the results of an EKG?

9. What do you like most about this career?

(Continued)

10. What advice would you have for others who want to do similar work?

____

____

11. What additional courses do you wish you had taken in high school or college?

____

____

12. What medical terms or abbreviations do you commonly use?

____

____

Part 2

After the Clinical Experience

Instructions: For each item below, identify whether you observed or assisted. Then, provide a brief summary.

Orientation

1. Client assessment
   - ☐ Observed
   - ☐ Assisted

   Brief summary:

   ____

   ____

2. Emergency procedures
   - ☐ Observed
   - ☐ Assisted

   Brief summary:

   ____

   ____

Non-Invasive Procedures

3. 12-lead EKG
   - ☐ Observed
   - ☐ Assisted

   Brief summary:

   ____

   ____

(Continued)

Name ____________________

4. Identification of EKG patterns (normal and arrhythmias)
   ☐ Observed
   ☐ Assisted
   Brief summary:
   ____
   ____

5. Telemetry monitors
   ☐ Observed
   ☐ Assisted
   Brief summary:
   ____
   ____

6. Stress test (List method observed)
   ☐ Observed
   ☐ Assisted
   Brief summary:
   ____
   ____

7. Pulse oximeters
   ☐ Observed
   ☐ Assisted
   Brief summary:
   ____
   ____

8. Holter monitor
   ☐ Observed
   ☐ Assisted
   Brief summary:
   ____
   ____

9. Echocardiogram
   ☐ Observed
   ☐ Assisted
   Brief summary:
   ____
   ____

(Continued)

10. Defibrillators
    ☐ Observed
    ☐ Assisted
    Brief summary:

    ____

    ____

11. Cardioversion
    ☐ Observed
    ☐ Assisted
    Brief summary:

    ____

    ____

12. Cardiac rehabilitation
    ☐ Observed
    ☐ Assisted
    Brief summary:

    ____

    ____

Invasive Procedures

13. Heart catheter
    ☐ Observed
    ☐ Assisted
    Brief summary:

    ____

    ____

14. Stent (PTCA)
    ☐ Observed
    ☐ Assisted
    Brief summary:

    ____

    ____

15. Pacemaker
    ☐ Observed
    ☐ Assisted
    Brief summary:

    ____

    ____

(Continued)

Name ______________________________

16. Coronary artery bypass graft
    - ☐ Observed
    - ☐ Assisted

    Brief summary:

    ____

    ____

17. Endarterectomy
    - ☐ Observed
    - ☐ Assisted

    Brief summary:

    ____

    ____

Student Name: ______________________________

Technician Name: ______________________________

Notes

Student ____________ Dates ____________ Site ____________ Preceptor ____________

Cardiopulmonary Post-Clinical Reflection

Rotation Report

Overview

Instructions: Answer the following questions using complete sentences.

1. What were your responsibilities or duties this week?

____

____

2. What new knowledge or skill did you learn or observe this week?

____

____

3. What was the best thing that happened at your clinical site this week?

____

____

4. What was the most challenging thing that happened at your clinical site this week?

____

____

5. What problems or difficulties did you encounter or observe at your clinical site? How were they dealt with?

____

____

6. Was this week good, fair, or bad? Explain.

____

____

Observations

Instructions: List the observations you made for each of the following categories.

1. Technology observed:

____

____

2. Diagnostic procedures observed:

____

____

(Continued)

3. Therapeutic procedures observed:

4. Diseases or disorders observed:

5. Medical terminology or abbreviations encountered:

6. Other observations:

Supervisor Signature: ______________________

Date: ______________________

Rotation Journal

Instructions: Write a journal entry detailing your learning experience at the clinical rotation. Use the following topics to help write a complete journal entry.

Assessment of the Environment

- Personnel
- Services provided
- Equipment
- Technology utilized

Observation

- Health care providers
- Team skills
- Communication skills
- Safety procedures
- Therapeutic/diagnostic procedures

Knowledge

- New information learned
- Medical terminology
- Skills learned

Evaluation

- Personal experience
- Educational value
- Professional value

Journal Entry

Write a journal entry summarizing your clinical experience.

Name ______________________ Date ____________ Period ____________

Dental Pre-Clinical Worksheet

Instructions: Answer the following questions.

1. How many baby teeth does the average person have?

___

2. How many permanent teeth does the average person have?

___

3. What is another name for the *third molars* and how many does the average person have?

___

___

4. Define the following:

A. Primary teeth:

___

___

B. Secondary teeth:

___

___

C. Incisors teeth:

___

___

D. Canine teeth:

___

___

E. Bicuspids teeth:

___

___

F. Molars teeth:

___

___

G. Impacted:

___

___

(Continued)

H. Dental caries:

I. Halitosis:

J. Canker sore:

K. Periodontal disease:

L. Gingivitis:

M. Scurvy:

N. Bruxism:

O. Dental abscess:

P. Leukoplakia:

Q. Dry socket:

R. Enamel:

S. Mandible:

(Continued)

Name ____________________

T. Maxilla:

____

____

U. Root canal:

____

____

5. Describe the function of the following:

A. Sublingual gland

____

____

B. Tongue

____

____

6. Research one disorder (cleft lip, cleft palate, or oral cancer) and record the following information.

A. Disorder

____

B. Symptoms

____

____

C. Etiology

____

____

D. Diagnosis

____

____

E. Treatment

____

____

F. Prognosis with and without treatment

____

____

(Continued)

Notes

Name ______________________ Date ____________ Period ____________

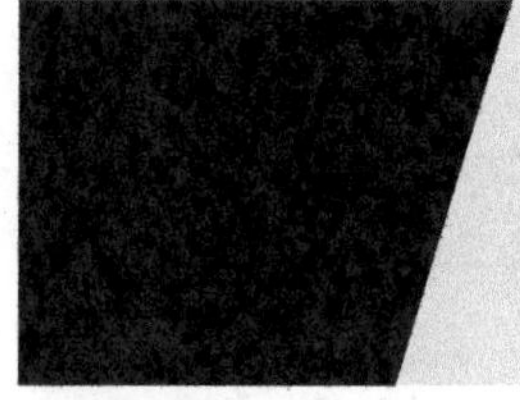

Dental Workplace Discovery Sheet

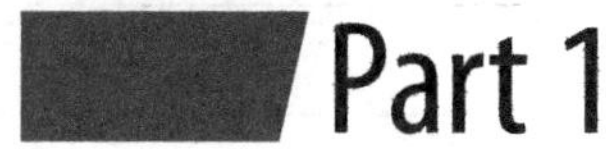

Part 1

During the Clinical Experience

Instructions: Answer the following questions.

1. What does a dental laboratory technician do?

2. What education and training are necessary to work as a dental laboratory technician?

3. What professionals work in the dental office?

4. What is the procedure for preparing the client for the doctor or hygienist?

5. What is the procedure followed when performing dental X-rays?

6. What types of anesthetics are commonly used for pulling or filling a tooth?

7. What types of materials are commonly used for filling a tooth?

8. What client education is done during a routine cleaning?

(Continued)

9. What type of training is required to become an oral surgeon? An orthodontist?

10. How are oral surgery or orthodontic procedures determined?

11. Why is it important to straighten teeth?

12. What happens during a root canal?

13. What does an impaction of a tooth mean?

14. What are the types of careers and educational requirements needed for the professionals who work in a prosthodontics office?

15. Are there any challenges related to the practice in prosthodontics?

16. What is the average number of clients seen daily in the clinic?

17. What is the most common condition seen in the clinic? What is the most challenging condition to treat?

18. What does a normal day look like in this profession?

(Continued)

Name ______________________________

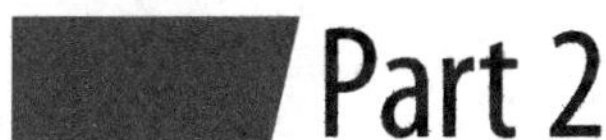

Part 2

After the Clinical Experience

Instructions: For each item below, identify whether you observed or assisted. Then, provide a brief summary.

Orientation and Safety

1. OSHA binder
   ☐ Observed
   ☐ Assisted
   Brief summary:
   ____
   ____

2. SDS labeling
   ☐ Observed
   ☐ Assisted
   Brief summary:
   ____
   ____

3. Infection control
   ☐ Observed
   ☐ Assisted
   Brief summary:
   ____
   ____

Equipment and Supplies

4. Dental lathes
   ☐ Observed
   ☐ Assisted
   Brief summary:
   ____
   ____

5. Dental engines
   ☐ Observed
   ☐ Assisted
   Brief summary:
   ____
   ____

(Continued)

6. Dental vibrators
   - ☐ Observed
   - ☐ Assisted

   Brief summary:

   ____

   ____

7. Dental stones
   - ☐ Observed
   - ☐ Assisted

   Brief summary:

   ____

   ____

8. Burnout and porcelain ovens
   - ☐ Observed
   - ☐ Assisted

   Brief summary:

   ____

   ____

9. Casting machines and torches
   - ☐ Observed
   - ☐ Assisted

   Brief summary:

   ____

   ____

Instruments

10. Needle holders
    - ☐ Observed
    - ☐ Assisted

    Brief summary:

    ____

    ____

11. Suture scissors
    - ☐ Observed
    - ☐ Assisted

    Brief summary:

    ____

    ____

(Continued)

Name ____________________

12. Periosteal elevators
    - ☐ Observed
    - ☐ Assisted

    Brief summary:

    ____

    ____

13. Rongiers
    - ☐ Observed
    - ☐ Assisted

    Brief summary:

    ____

    ____

14. Extraction forceps
    - ☐ Observed
    - ☐ Assisted

    Brief summary:

    ____

    ____

15. Surgical aspirator tips observed
    - ☐ Observed
    - ☐ Assisted

    Brief summary:

    ____

    ____

16. Root tip picks
    - ☐ Observed
    - ☐ Assisted

    Brief summary:

    ____

    ____

17. Minnesota retractor
    - ☐ Observed
    - ☐ Assisted

    Brief summary:

    ____

    ____

(Continued)

18. Mirror
    ☐ Observed
    ☐ Assisted
    Brief summary:

    ____

    ____

19. Lip retractors
    ☐ Observed
    ☐ Assisted
    Brief summary:

    ____

    ____

20. Cotton pliers
    ☐ Observed
    ☐ Assisted
    Brief summary:

    ____

    ____

21. Hemostat
    ☐ Observed
    ☐ Assisted
    Brief summary:

    ____

    ____

22. Scaler
    ☐ Observed
    ☐ Assisted
    Brief summary:

    ____

    ____

23. Tucker
    ☐ Observed
    ☐ Assisted
    Brief summary:

    ____

    ____

(Continued)

Name ______________________________

24. Explorer
   - ☐ Observed
   - ☐ Assisted

   Brief summary:

   ____

   ____

25. Spatula
   - ☐ Observed
   - ☐ Assisted

   Brief summary:

   ____

   ____

26. Pliers
   - ☐ Observed
   - ☐ Assisted

   Brief summary:

   ____

   ____

Dental Laboratory Procedures

27. Fabrication of various custom trays
   - ☐ Observed
   - ☐ Assisted

   Brief summary:

   ____

   ____

28. Pouring and mounting master cast
   - ☐ Observed
   - ☐ Assisted

   Brief summary:

   ____

   ____

29. Full crowns
   - ☐ Observed
   - ☐ Assisted

   Brief summary:

   ____

   ____

(Continued)

30. Fixed bridges
    ☐ Observed
    ☐ Assisted
    Brief summary:

    ___

    ___

31. Dentures
    ☐ Observed
    ☐ Assisted
    Brief summary:

    ___

    ___

Routine Dental Visits

32. Client seating, draping, and positioning
    ☐ Observed
    ☐ Assisted
    Brief summary:

    ___

    ___

33. Dental charting (DMF)
    ☐ Observed
    ☐ Assisted
    Brief summary:

    ___

    ___

34. Dental radiology (FMX Panoramic)
    ☐ Observed
    ☐ Assisted
    Brief summary:

    ___

    ___

35. Oral hygiene instruction
    ☐ Observed
    ☐ Assisted
    Brief summary:

    ___

    ___

(Continued)

Name ____________________

36. Dental prophylaxis
    ☐ Observed
    ☐ Assisted
    Brief summary:

    ____

    ____

37. Discharge instructions
    ☐ Observed
    ☐ Assisted
    Brief summary:

    ____

    ____

Chairside Assisting

38. Selection of appropriate dental tray
    ☐ Observed
    ☐ Assisted
    Brief summary:

    ____

    ____

39. Loading anesthetic syringe
    ☐ Observed
    ☐ Assisted
    Brief summary:

    ____

    ____

40. Monitoring N2O
    ☐ Observed
    ☐ Assisted
    Brief summary:

    ____

    ____

41. Prep of various materials
    ☐ Observed
    ☐ Assisted
    Brief summary:

    ____

    ____

(Continued)

42. Passing of dental instruments
☐ Observed
☐ Assisted
Brief summary:

____

____

43. Suctioning
☐ Observed
☐ Assisted
Brief summary:

____

____

44. Discharge instructions
☐ Observed
☐ Assisted
Brief summary:

____

____

45. Client monitors
☐ Observed
☐ Assisted
Brief summary:

____

____

46. Sterile field
☐ Observed
☐ Assisted
Brief summary:

____

____

47. Extractions
☐ Observed
☐ Assisted
Brief summary:

____

____

(Continued)

Name ______________________________

48. Biopsy
   - ☐ Observed
   - ☐ Assisted

   Brief summary:

   ____

   ____

49. Suture placement
   - ☐ Observed
   - ☐ Assisted

   Brief summary:

   ____

   ____

50. Alveoloplasty
   - ☐ Observed
   - ☐ Assisted

   Brief summary:

   ____

   ____

51. Implant placement
   - ☐ Observed
   - ☐ Assisted

   Brief summary:

   ____

   ____

52. Periodontal surgery
   - ☐ Observed
   - ☐ Assisted

   Brief summary:

   ____

   ____

53. Separators
   - ☐ Observed
   - ☐ Assisted

   Brief summary:

   ____

   ____

(Continued)

54. Brackets and molar bands

☐ Observed

☐ Assisted

Brief summary:

____

____

55. Change elastomeric ties and archwires

☐ Observed

☐ Assisted

Brief summary:

____

____

56. Coil springs and power chain

☐ Observed

☐ Assisted

Brief summary:

____

____

57. Retainers

☐ Observed

☐ Assisted

Brief summary:

____

____

58. Periosteal elevators

☐ Observed

☐ Assisted

Brief summary:

____

____

59. Rongiers

☐ Observed

☐ Assisted

Brief summary:

____

____

(Continued)

Name ______________________________

Operative Procedures

60. Diagnostic impressions/models
    - ☐ Observed
    - ☐ Assisted

    Brief summary:

    ____

    ____

61. Restorative
    - ☐ Observed
    - ☐ Assisted

    Brief summary:

    ____

    ____

62. Cosmetics
    - ☐ Observed
    - ☐ Assisted

    Brief summary:

    ____

    ____

63. Prosthetics
    - ☐ Observed
    - ☐ Assisted

    Brief summary:

    ____

    ____

Student Name: ______________________________

Technician Name: ______________________________

Notes

Student ______________________ Dates __________ Site __________ Preceptor __________

Dental Post-Clinical Reflection

Rotation Report

Overview

Instructions: Answer the following questions using complete sentences.

1. What were your responsibilities or duties this week?

____

____

2. What new knowledge or skill did you learn or observe this week?

____

____

3. What was the best thing that happened at your clinical site this week?

____

____

4. What was the most challenging thing that happened at your clinical site this week?

____

____

5. What problems or difficulties did you encounter or observe at your clinical site? How were they dealt with?

____

____

6. Was this week good, fair, or bad? Explain.

____

____

Observations

Instructions: List the observations you made for each of the following categories.

1. Technology observed:

____

____

2. Diagnostic procedures observed:

____

____

(Continued)

3. Therapeutic procedures observed:

4. Diseases or disorders observed:

5. Medical terminology or abbreviations encountered:

6. Other observations:

Supervisor Signature: ______________________________

Date: ______________________________

Rotation Journal

Instructions: Write a journal entry detailing your learning experience at the clinical rotation. Use the following topics to help write a complete journal entry.

Assessment of the Environment

- Personnel
- Services provided
- Equipment
- Technology utilized

Observation

- Health care providers
- Team skills
- Communication skills
- Safety procedures
- Therapeutic/diagnostic procedures

Knowledge

- New information learned
- Medical terminology
- Skills learned

Evaluation

- Personal experience
- Educational value
- Professional value

Journal Entry

Write a journal entry summarizing your clinical experience.

Name ______________________ Date ____________ Period ____________

Digestive and Nutrition Pre-Clinical Worksheet

Instructions: Answer the following questions.

1. Label the parts of the digestive system.

A. ______________________

B. ______________________

C. ______________________

D. ______________________

E. ______________________

F. ______________________

G. ______________________

H. ______________________

I. ______________________

J. ______________________

K. ______________________

L. ______________________

M. ______________________

N. ______________________

O. ______________________

P. ______________________

Q. ______________________

R. ______________________

S. ______________________

T. ______________________

U. ______________________

V. ______________________

W. ______________________

X. ______________________

Y. ______________________

© *Body Scientific International*

(Continued)

2. Identify and describe six essential nutrients your body needs.

3. Describe the following functions of the digestive system.

A. Ingestion:

B. Digestion:

C. Absorption:

D. Elimination:

4. Describe the following pancreatic excretions:

A. Amylase:

B. Lipase:

C. Protease:

D. Insulin:

5. Differentiate between saturated and unsaturated lipids.

6. Describe the difference between HDL, LDL, and triglycerides.

(Continued)

Name ____________________

7. When digested, what are fats, proteins, and carbohydrates broken down into?
   A. Fats:
   ____
   B. Proteins:
   ____
   C. Carbohydrates:
   ____

8. Where does most nutrient absorption occur in the digestive system (be specific)?
   ____
   ____

9. Describe the difference between a fat-soluble vitamin and a water-soluble vitamin.
   ____
   ____

10. Explain the difference between a vitamin and a mineral.
   ____
   ____

11. List the solubility, function, food source, and daily requirements for each of the following vitamins and minerals.
   A. Vitamin A:
   ____
   ____
   B. Vitamin B12:
   ____
   ____
   C. Vitamin C:
   ____
   ____
   D. Vitamin D:
   ____
   ____
   E. Vitamin E:
   ____
   ____
   F. Vitamin K:
   ____
   ____

(Continued)

G. Niacin:

H. Folic acid:

I. Riboflavin:

J. Biotin:

K. Calcium:

12. Explain the importance of a normal intake-output balance.

13. What is a therapeutic diet?

14. Briefly describe the following therapeutic diets:
    A. Clear liquid

    B. Full liquid

    C. Low calorie

    D. Low carb

    E. Low fat

(Continued)

Name ____

F. Low cholesterol

____

____

G. Low residue

____

____

H. Diabetic

____

____

I. High protein

____

____

15. Define hyperalimentation.

____

____

16. Give examples of when a tube feeding would be ordered.

____

____

17. Identify four common symptoms of a food-borne illness

____

____

18. Identify two common bacteria and two common parasites that cause food-borne illness.

Bacteria:

____

Parasites:

____

Notes

Name ______________________ Date ____________ Period ____________

Digestive and Nutrition Workplace Discovery Sheet

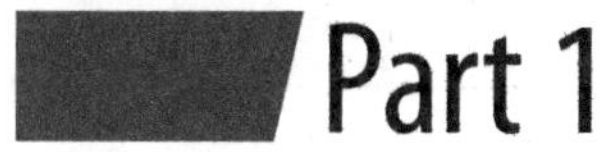

Part 1

During the Clinical Experience

Instructions: Answer the following questions.

1. On a typical day, how many different types of diets are needed?

____

____

2. What percentage of clients will this department be required to spend in person time on educating about their dietary needs?

____

____

3. What disorders/diets do you spend the most time educating clients on?

____

____

4. Who is responsible for checking food trays leaving the dietary department?

____

____

5. Who delivers the tray to clients on the floor and what communication is standard with the nursing unit?

____

____

6. For clients who require tube feeding, who decides on what nutrients to give and who makes it?

____

____

7. Can clients with feeding tubes still eat by mouth?

____

____

8. What are some of the complications associated with a feeding tube?

____

____

(Continued)

9. What circumstances may cause a client to need a feeding tube?

10. List the entrance point, target client, pros, and cons for each of the following types of feeding tubes.
    A. Nasogastric (NG):
    B. Nasojejunal (NJT):
    C. Jejunostomy (JEJ):
    D. Radiologically inserted tube (RIG):
    E. Percutaneous endoscopic gastronomy tube (PEG):

11. Mr. Smith is a client who experienced a heart attack last week. The next day, he underwent coronary artery bypass grafting (CABG). Before being released, dietary was asked to help him understand the new diet he should be on after leaving the hospital. The doctor has requested a consultation for a low sodium, low cholesterol, low calorie diet. What are some examples of food he can eat for each meal? What are the suggested servings?
    A. Breakfast:
    B. Lunch:
    C. Snack:
    D. Dinner:

(Continued)

Name ______________________________

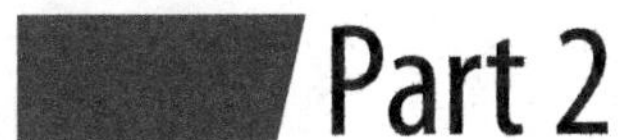

Part 2

After the Clinical Experience

Instructions: For each item below, identify whether you observed or assisted. Then, provide a brief summary.

Awareness of Relation Between Food and Health

1. Body's use of nutrients
   - ☐ Observed
   - ☐ Assisted

   Brief summary:

   ____

   ____

2. Dietary guidelines through life stages
   - ☐ Observed
   - ☐ Assisted

   Brief summary:

   ____

   ____

3. Food customs
   - ☐ Observed
   - ☐ Assisted

   Brief summary:

   ____

   ____

Management of Dietary Services

4. Sanitary and safety rules
   - ☐ Observed
   - ☐ Assisted

   Brief summary:

   ____

   ____

5. Purchase of food
   - ☐ Observed
   - ☐ Assisted

   Brief summary:

   ____

   ____

(Continued)

6. Special equipment
   ☐ Observed
   ☐ Assisted
   Brief summary:

   ____

   ____

Dietary Services

7. Plan menus
   ☐ Observed
   ☐ Assisted
   Brief summary:

   ____

   ____

8. Help clients select menus
   ☐ observed
   ☐ Assisted
   Brief summary:

   ____

   ____

9. Distribution of foods
   ☐ Observed
   ☐ Assisted
   Brief summary:

   ____

   ____

Special Diets

10. Nutritional assessment and therapy
    ☐ Observed
    ☐ Assisted
    Brief summary:

    ____

    ____

11. Diseases/Disorders requiring intervention
    ☐ Observed
    ☐ Assisted
    Brief summary:

    ____

    ____

(Continued)

Name ____________________

12. Client education
    ☐ Observed
    ☐ Assisted
    Brief summary:
    ____
    ____

13. Weight management
    ☐ Observed
    ☐ Assisted
    Brief summary:
    ____
    ____

Special Considerations

14. Diabetes
    ☐ Observed
    ☐ Assisted
    Brief summary:
    ____
    ____

15. Cardiovascular disease
    ☐ Observed
    ☐ Assisted
    Brief summary:
    ____
    ____

16. Cancer, surgery, burns, infection
    ☐ Observed
    ☐ Assisted
    Brief summary:
    ____
    ____

Student Name: ____________________

Technician Name: ____________________

Notes

Student ______________________ Dates __________ Site __________ Preceptor __________

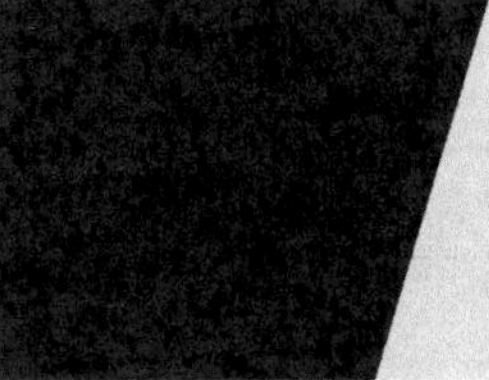

Digestive and Nutrition Post-Clinical Reflection

Rotation Report

Overview

Instructions: Answer the following questions using complete sentences.

1. What were your responsibilities or duties this week?

____

____

2. What new knowledge or skill did you learn or observe this week?

____

____

3. What was the best thing that happened at your clinical site this week?

____

____

4. What was the most challenging thing that happened at your clinical site this week?

____

____

5. What problems or difficulties did you encounter or observe at your clinical site? How were they dealt with?

____

____

6. Was this week good, fair, or bad? Explain.

____

____

Observations

Instructions: List the observations you made for each of the following categories.

1. Technology observed:

____

____

2. Diagnostic procedures observed:

____

____

(Continued)

3. Therapeutic procedures observed:

____

____

4. Diseases or disorders observed:

____

____

5. Medical terminology or abbreviations encountered:

____

____

6. Other observations:

____

____

Supervisor Signature: ______________________________

Date: ______________________________

Rotation Journal

Instructions: Write a journal entry detailing your learning experience at the clinical rotation. Use the following topics to help write a complete journal entry.

Assessment of the Environment

- Personnel
- Services provided
- Equipment
- Technology utilized

Observation

- Health care providers
- Team skills
- Communication skills
- Safety procedures
- Therapeutic/diagnostic procedures

Knowledge

- New information learned
- Medical terminology
- Skills learned

Evaluation

- Personal experience
- Educational value
- Professional value

Journal Entry

Write a journal entry summarizing your clinical experience.

____

____

____

____

____

____

Name ______________________ Date ____________ Period ____________

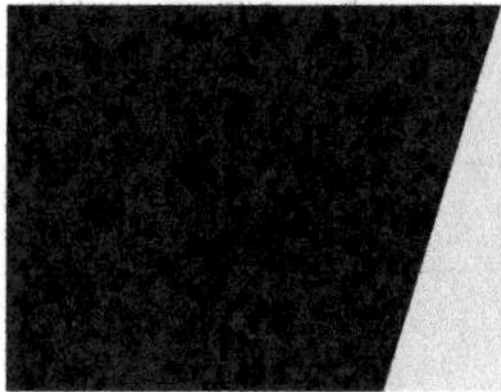

Emergency Services Pre-Clinical Worksheet

Instructions: Answer the following questions.

1. Define the following terms and conditions:
   A. Hypovolemic shock:

   ____

   ____

   B. Septic shock:

   ____

   ____

   C. Neurogenic shock:

   ____

   ____

   D. Anaphylactic shock:

   ____

   ____

   E. Psychogenic shock:

   ____

   ____

   F. Respiratory failure:

   ____

   ____

   G. COPD:

   ____

   ____

   H. Cardiac failure:

   ____

   ____

   I. Multisystem trauma:

   ____

   ____

   J. Nature of illness (NOI):

   ____

   ____

(Continued)

K. Mechanism of injury (MOI):

2. What are the signs and symptoms of a stroke?

3. What is a transient ischemic attack (TIA) and does it require treatment?

4. Briefly explain the etiology of each of the four common types of seizures.

A. Epileptic:

B. Structural:

C. Metabolic:

D. Febrile:

5. What are the four common ways a person may be poisoned?

6. What are the two common types of sugar emergencies seen by emergency personnel and how do you treat them?

7. What is the Glasgow Trauma Score and how is it calculated?

8. What does the rule of nines help emergency staff evaluate?

(Continued)

Name ______________________________

9. What is the difference between a laceration and an avulsion?

10. What is urticaria and how is it treated?

11. What is the difference between a concussion and a contusion on the brain?

12. Define the following orthopedic injuries.
    A. Dislocation:

    B. Sprain:

    C. Strains:

    D. Open fracture:

    E. Closed fracture:

    F. Compartment syndrome:

    G. Amputation:

    H. RICE:

(Continued)

13. Look up the following respiratory disorders, then record their etiology and preferred treatment.

A. Asthma:

____

____

B. Bronchitis:

____

____

C. Congestive heart failure:

____

____

D. COVID:

____

____

E. Croup:

____

____

F. Emphysema:

____

____

G. Pneumonia:

____

____

H. Pneumothorax:

____

____

I. Pulmonary embolus:

____

____

J. Pertussis:

____

____

Name ______________________ Date ____________ Period ____________

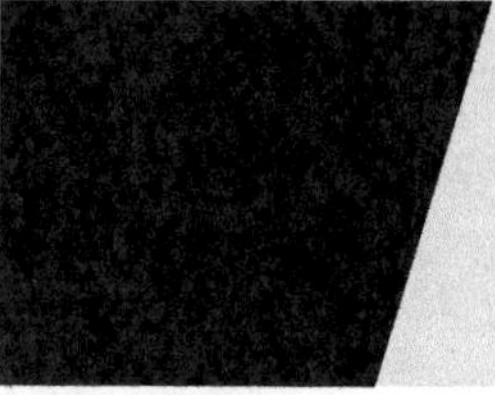

Emergency Services Workplace Discovery Sheet

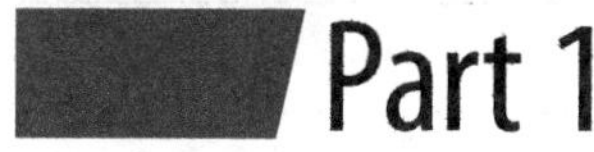

Part 1

During the Clinical Experience

Instructions: Answer the following questions.

1. What is triage? Describe the process.

2. List the equipment found in a standard client emergency room.

3. List additional equipment found in a trauma room that was not in a standard client emergency room.

4. Where are the emergency medications kept?

5. What is the difference between a defibrillator and an AED?

6. What types of emergencies are brought back immediately?

7. Name a procedure that you were surprised that clients came to the emergency room for.

8. During what part of client assessment does the EMS determine the client priority of care and transport?

(Continued)

9. List the equipment found in a standard EMS vehicle.

10. List four types of clients who are classified as "load and go."

11. Emergency personnel are trained for mass casualty situations. What do the following colors mean in this context?
    A. Green:
    B. Yellow:
    C. Red:
    D. Black:

12. What are the following emergency medications used for out in the field?
    A. Nitroglycerin:
    B. Epinephrine:
    C. NARCAN:

13. What type of clients are placed on a back board?

14. List three methods commonly used to give the client oxygen out in the field.

15. Even though the client is critical, why may the ambulance not use its lights and sirens when headed to the ER?

16. What is involved with handing off the client to the ER?

(Continued)

Name ____

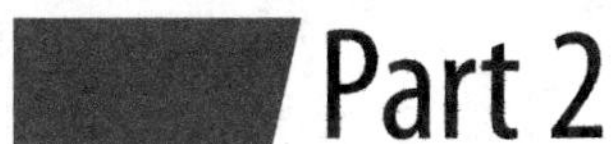

Part 2

After the Clinical Experience

Instructions: For each item below, identify whether you observed or assisted. Then, provide a brief summary.

Orientation

1. Emergency department

   ☐ Observed

   ☐ Assisted

   Brief summary:

   ____

   ____

2. Ambulance/Fire truck

   ☐ Observed

   ☐ Assisted

   Brief summary:

   ____

   ____

Triage

3. Primary assessment

   ☐ Observed

   ☐ Assisted

   Brief summary:

   ____

   ____

4. Secondary assessment

   ☐ Observed

   ☐ Assisted

   Brief summary:

   ____

   ____

5. Vital signs

   ☐ Observed

   ☐ Assisted

   Brief summary:

   ____

   ____

(Continued)

Treatments

6. Medical assessment
   ☐ Observed
   ☐ Assisted
   Brief summary:
   ____
   ____

7. Trauma assessment
   ☐ Observed
   ☐ Assisted
   Brief summary:
   ____
   ____

Special Procedures

8. EENT
   ☐ Observed
   ☐ Assisted
   Brief summary:
   ____
   ____

9. Obstetrics
   ☐ Observed
   ☐ Assisted
   Brief summary:
   ____
   ____

10. Radiography
   ☐ Observed
   ☐ Assisted
   Brief summary:
   ____
   ____

11. Laboratory
   ☐ Observed
   ☐ Assisted
   Brief summary:
   ____
   ____

(Continued)

Name ______________________________

12. IV
    - ☐ Observed
    - ☐ Assisted

    Brief summary:

    ____

    ____

13. Medication
    - ☐ Observed
    - ☐ Assisted

    Brief summary:

    ____

    ____

14. Spinal alignment
    - ☐ Observed
    - ☐ Assisted

    Brief summary:

    ____

    ____

15. Lifts and carries
    - ☐ Observed
    - ☐ Assisted

    Brief summary:

    ____

    ____

Student Name: ______________________________

Technician Name: ______________________________

Notes

Student ______________________ Dates ____________ Site ____________ Preceptor ____________

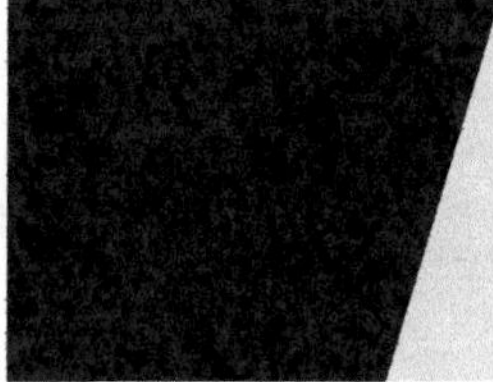

Emergency Services Post-Clinical Reflection

Rotation Report

Overview

Instructions: Answer the following questions using complete sentences.

1. What were your responsibilities or duties this week?

____

____

2. What new knowledge or skill did you learn or observe this week?

____

____

3. What was the best thing that happened at your clinical site this week?

____

____

4. What was the most challenging thing that happened at your clinical site this week?

____

____

5. What problems or difficulties did you encounter or observe at your clinical site? How were they dealt with?

____

____

6. Was this week good, fair, or bad? Explain.

____

____

Observations

Instructions: List the observations you made for each of the following categories.

1. Technology observed:

____

____

2. Diagnostic procedures observed:

____

____

(Continued)

3. Therapeutic procedures observed:

____

____

4. Diseases or disorders observed:

____

____

5. Medical terminology or abbreviations encountered:

____

____

6. Other observations:

____

____

Supervisor Signature: ____________________________

Date: ____________________________

Rotation Journal

Instructions: Write a journal entry detailing your learning experience at the clinical rotation. Use the following topics to help write a complete journal entry.

Assessment of the Environment

- Personnel
- Services provided
- Equipment
- Technology utilized

Observation

- Health care providers
- Team skills
- Communication skills
- Safety procedures
- Therapeutic/diagnostic procedures

Knowledge

- New information learned
- Medical terminology
- Skills learned

Evaluation

- Personal experience
- Educational value
- Professional value

Journal Entry

Write a journal entry summarizing your clinical experience.

____

____

____

____

____

____

Name ______________________ Date __________ Period __________

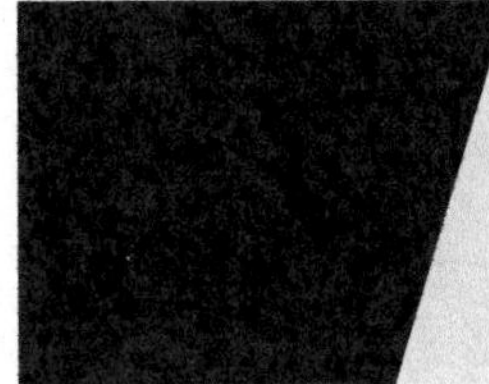

Endocrine Pre-Clinical Worksheet

Instructions: Answer the following questions.

1. What risk factors are associated with diabetes?

2. List the etiology and the common signs and symptoms for the following types of diabetes.

   A. Type 1 diabetes (juvenile):

   B. Type 2 diabetes (mellitus):

   C. Gestational diabetes:

   D. Maturity onset diabetes of the young (MODY):

   E. Neonatal diabetes:

   F. Wolfram Syndrome:

   G. Alstrom Syndrome:

   H. Latent autoimmune diabetes in adults (LADA):

   I. Steroid-induced diabetes:

(Continued)

3. What special procedures are part of the assessment for a client who has diabetes?

4. What type of lab work is monitored on someone diagnosed with diabetes?

5. What is a Hemoglobin A1C and what do the results mean?

6. What is the normal range for a blood glucose screening test?

7. Why is it important for people who have diabetes to see a podiatrist?

8. Define the following terms:

   A. Glaucoma:

   B. Hypoglycemia:

   C. Hyperglycemia:

   D. Hyperlipidemia:

   E. Hypertension:

   F. Neuropathy:

(Continued)

Name ____

G. Urine ketones:

____

____

H. Blood glucose meter:

____

____

I. Continuous glucose monitors:

____

____

J. Injection pens:

____

____

K. Insulin pumps:

____

____

L. Automated insulin delivery system:

____

____

Notes

Name ______________________ Date ____________ Period ____________

Endocrine Workplace Discovery Sheet

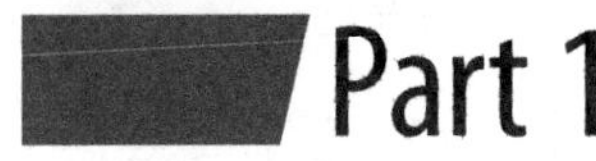

Part 1

During the Clinical Experience

Instructions: Answer the following questions.

1. What type of education or background do most of the staff have in this department?

2. Do you see mainly in-clients or out-clients?

3. Do you get referrals from doctors' offices?

4. What does follow-up look like with the clients for this department?

5. How do you educate clients on diets?

6. How do individual exercise programs work and what does that look like?

7. What different types of medication therapy do you use in this area?

8. Explain how an insulin pump works differently from insulin injections and the pros and cons of each.

(Continued)

9. What type of community resources referrals may be utilized by clients with diabetes?

____

____

Part 2

After the Clinical Experience

Instructions: For each item below, identify whether you observed or assisted. Then, provide a brief summary.

Orientation

1. Client assessment
   ☐ Observed
   ☐ Assisted
   Brief summary:

   ____

   ____

2. Emergency procedures
   ☐ Observed
   ☐ Assisted
   Brief summary:

   ____

   ____

Diet Therapy

3. Nutritional assessment
   ☐ Observed
   ☐ Assisted
   Brief summary:

   ____

   ____

4. Instructions on ADA diets
   ☐ Observed
   ☐ Assisted
   Brief summary:

   ____

   ____

(Continued)

Name ____

Exercise

5. Individual exercise plan
   - ☐ Observed
   - ☐ Assisted

   Brief summary:

   ____

   ____

6. Precautions during/after exercise
   - ☐ Observed
   - ☐ Assisted

   Brief summary:

   ____

   ____

Medication Therapy

7. Instruction on oral agents–action, timing
   - ☐ Observed
   - ☐ Assisted

   Brief summary:

   ____

   ____

8. Instruction on insulin administration–storage, action, timing
   - ☐ Observed
   - ☐ Assisted

   Brief summary:

   ____

   ____

9. Special considerations
   - ☐ Observed
   - ☐ Assisted

   Brief summary:

   ____

   ____

(Continued)

Complications

10. Hyperglycemia
    - ☐ Observed
    - ☐ Assisted

    Brief summary:

    ____

    ____

11. Hypoglycemia
    - ☐ Observed
    - ☐ Assisted

    Brief summary:

    ____

    ____

12. Chronic complications
    - ☐ Observed
    - ☐ Assisted

    Brief summary:

    ____

    ____

Glucose Monitoring

13. Rationale for monitoring
    - ☐ Observed
    - ☐ Assisted

    Brief summary:

    ____

    ____

14. Timing
    - ☐ Observed
    - ☐ Assisted

    Brief summary:

    ____

    ____

15. Instructions on glucose meter
    - ☐ Observed
    - ☐ Assisted

    Brief summary:

    ____

    ____

(Continued)

Name ______________________________

Gestational Diabetes Mellitus Management (GDM)

16. Consequences of hyperglycemia in GDM
    - ☐ Observed
    - ☐ Assisted

    Brief summary:

    ____

    ____

17. Self-management instructions
    - ☐ Observed
    - ☐ Assisted

    Brief summary:

    ____

    ____

Other

18. Community resources
    - ☐ Observed
    - ☐ Assisted

    Brief summary:

    ____

    ____

Student Name: ______________________________

Technician Name: ______________________________

Notes

Student ______________________ Dates ____________ Site ____________ Preceptor ____________

Endocrine Post-Clinical Reflection

Rotation Report

Overview

Instructions: Answer the following questions using complete sentences.

1. What were your responsibilities or duties this week?

____

____

2. What new knowledge or skill did you learn or observe this week?

____

____

3. What was the best thing that happened at your clinical site this week?

____

____

4. What was the most challenging thing that happened at your clinical site this week?

____

____

5. What problems or difficulties did you encounter or observe at your clinical site? How were they dealt with?

____

____

6. Was this week good, fair, or bad? Explain.

____

____

Observations

Instructions: List the observations you made for each of the following categories.

1. Technology observed:

____

____

2. Diagnostic procedures observed:

____

____

(Continued)

3. Therapeutic procedures observed:

4. Diseases or disorders observed:

5. Medical terminology or abbreviations encountered:

6. Other observations:

Supervisor Signature: ____________________

Date: ____________________

Rotation Journal

Instructions: Write a journal entry detailing your learning experience at the clinical rotation. Use the following topics to help write a complete journal entry.

Assessment of the Environment

- Personnel
- Services provided
- Equipment
- Technology utilized

Observation

- Health care providers
- Team skills
- Communication skills
- Safety procedures
- Therapeutic/diagnostic procedures

Knowledge

- New information learned
- Medical terminology
- Skills learned

Evaluation

- Personal experience
- Educational value
- Professional value

Journal Entry

Write a journal entry summarizing your clinical experience.

Name ______________________ Date ____________ Period ____________

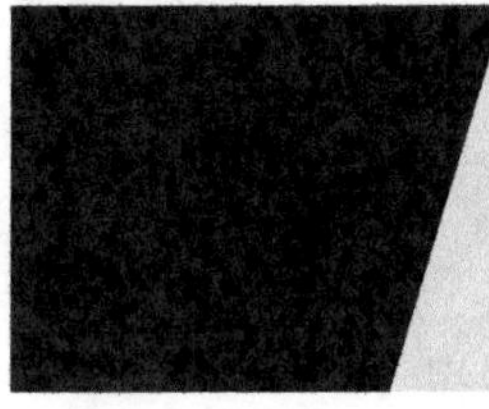

Geriatrics Pre-Clinical Worksheet

Instructions: Answer the following questions.

1. Describe three physiological changes that commonly occur in each body system with the aging process.

   A. Integumentary:

   B. Skeletal:

   C. Muscular:

   D. Sensory:

   E. Endocrine:

   F. Cardiovascular:

   G. Immune/Lymphatic:

   H. Respiratory:

   I. Gastrointestinal:

   J. Urinary:

(Continued)

K. Reproductive:

2. What are ADLs?

3. Define the following terms:

A. Kyphosis:

B. Arcus senilis:

C. Presbyopia:

D. Macular degeneration:

E. Glaucoma:

F. Cataracts:

G. Incontinence:

H. Dysphagia:

I. Neuropathy:

(Continued)

Name ______________________________

J. Dysphasia:

____

____

K. Vertigo:

____

____

4. Define the following age-related conditions, then list ADLs that might be affected by these conditions.

A. Coronary artery disease:

____

____

B. Ischemic stroke:

____

____

C. Hemorrhagic stroke:

____

____

D. Hypertension:

____

____

E. Type 2 diabetes:

____

____

F. Parkinson's disease:

____

____

G. Dementia:

____

____

H. Alzheimer's:

____

____

I. COPD:

____

____

J. Osteoarthritis:

____

____

(Continued)

K. Osteoporosis:

5. What types of cancer are common in older adult clients?

Name ______________________ Date ____________ Period __________

Geriatrics Workplace Discovery Sheet

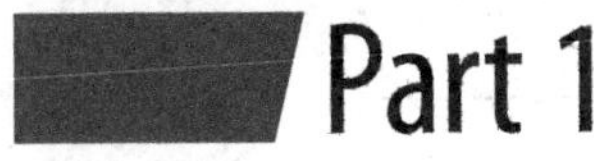

Part 1

During the Clinical Experience

Instructions: Answer the following questions.

1. List four reasons a client could be considered a fall risk.

2. What actions can you take to help prevent a client from falling?

3. When should you use a gait belt?

4. What is an adaptive device?

5. Name five adaptive devices used to help residents stay more independent and help to prevent falls.

6. What is a restraint and when can it be used?

7. What rules need to be followed when using a restraint?

8. Define ROM and describe the terms below related to ROM:

   A. Definition of ROM:

(Continued)

B. Extension:

C. Flexion:

D. Internal rotation:

E. External rotation:

F. Abduction:

G. Adduction:

9. How often should a client who is bedridden be turned?

10. Define the following terms:

A. Aphasia:

B. Atrophy:

C. Contracture:

D. Cyanotic:

(Continued)

Name ______________________________

E. Debilitating:

F. Deteriorated:

G. Decubitus ulcer:

H. Edema:

I. Foot drop:

J. Orthostatic hypotension:

K. Pallor:

L. Syncope:

M. Tenting:

11. What are some common methods used to turn or move a client in bed?

12. What is an intake and output form used for?

13. When emptying a foley catheter bag, what can you use to measure the amount of urine collected?

(Continued)

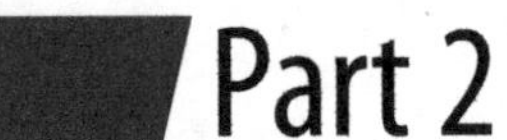 Part 2

After the Clinical Experience

Instructions: For each item below, identify whether you observed or assisted. Then, provide a brief summary.

Introduction to Long-Term Care

1. Handwashing
   ☐ Observed
   ☐ Assisted
   Brief summary:
   ____
   ____

2. Communication
   ☐ Observed
   ☐ Assisted
   Brief summary:
   ____
   ____

3. Clients with vision loss
   ☐ Observed
   ☐ Assisted
   Brief summary:
   ____
   ____

4. Clients with hearing loss
   ☐ Observed
   ☐ Assisted
   Brief summary:
   ____
   ____

5. Clients with speech issues
   ☐ Observed
   ☐ Assisted
   Brief summary:
   ____
   ____

(Continued)

Name ____

Mental Health and Social Services

6. Psychosocial needs of clients
   - ☐ Observed
   - ☐ Assisted

   Brief summary:

   ____

   ____

7. Clients with memory loss/confusion
   - ☐ Observed
   - ☐ Assisted

   Brief summary:

   ____

   ____

8. Clients who are demanding/angry
   - ☐ Observed
   - ☐ Assisted

   Brief summary:

   ____

   ____

Restorative Services

9. Assist clients to raise head/shoulder
   - ☐ Observed
   - ☐ Assisted

   Brief summary:

   ____

   ____

10. Assist clients to move up in bed
    - ☐ Observed
    - ☐ Assisted

    Brief summary:

    ____

    ____

11. Moving the client to the HOB
    - ☐ Observed
    - ☐ Assisted

    Brief summary:

    ____

    ____

(Continued)

12. Turning client on side
   - ☐ Observed
   - ☐ Assisted

   Brief summary:

   ___

   ___

13. Assist clients to sit on side of bed
   - ☐ Observed
   - ☐ Assisted

   Brief summary:

   ___

   ___

14. Assist clients to transfer to wheelchair
   - ☐ Observed
   - ☐ Assisted

   Brief summary:

   ___

   ___

15. Range-of-motion exercises
   - ☐ Observed
   - ☐ Assisted

   Brief summary:

   ___

   ___

16. Assist a client to ambulate with a walker
   - ☐ Observed
   - ☐ Assisted

   Brief summary:

   ___

   ___

Personal Care Skills

17. Making the unoccupied bed
   - ☐ Observed
   - ☐ Assisted

   Brief summary:

   ___

   ___

(Continued)

Name ______________________________

18. Making the occupied bed
    ☐ Observed
    ☐ Assisted
    Brief summary:
    ____
    ____

19. Tub or shower
    ☐ Observed
    ☐ Assisted
    Brief summary:
    ____
    ____

20. Partial bath
    ☐ Observed
    ☐ Assisted
    Brief summary:
    ____
    ____

21. Complete bed bath
    ☐ Observed
    ☐ Assisted
    Brief summary:
    ____
    ____

22. Perineal care female/male
    ☐ Observed
    ☐ Assisted
    Brief summary:
    ____
    ____

23. Backrub
    ☐ Observed
    ☐ Assisted
    Brief summary:
    ____
    ____

(Continued)

24. Brushing the teeth
☐ Observed
☐ Assisted
Brief summary:

____

____

25. Denture care
☐ Observed
☐ Assisted
Brief summary:

____

____

26. Special oral hygiene
☐ Observed
☐ Assisted
Brief summary:

____

____

27. Hair care
☐ Observed
☐ Assisted
Brief summary:

____

____

28. Shaving using an electric or safety razor
☐ Observed
☐ Assisted
Brief summary:

____

____

29. Hand and fingernail care
☐ Observed
☐ Assisted
Brief summary:

____

____

(Continued)

Name ____

30. Foot and toenail care

☐ Observed

☐ Assisted

Brief summary:

____

____

31. Assisting the client with dressing

☐ Observed

☐ Assisted

Brief summary:

____

____

32. Assisting the client with feeding

☐ Observed

☐ Assisted

Brief summary:

____

____

Student Name: ______________________________

Technician Name: ___________________________

Notes

Student ______________________ Dates ____________ Site ____________ Preceptor ____________

Geriatrics Post-Clinical Reflection

Rotation Report

Overview

Instructions: Answer the following questions using complete sentences.

1. What were your responsibilities or duties this week?

____

____

2. What new knowledge or skill did you learn or observe this week?

____

____

3. What was the best thing that happened at your clinical site this week?

____

____

4. What was the most challenging thing that happened at your clinical site this week?

____

____

5. What problems or difficulties did you encounter or observe at your clinical site? How were they dealt with?

____

____

6. Was this week good, fair, or bad? Explain.

____

____

Observations

Instructions: List the observations you made for each of the following categories.

1. Technology observed:

____

____

2. Diagnostic procedures observed:

____

____

(Continued)

3. Therapeutic procedures observed:

____

____

4. Diseases or disorders observed:

____

____

5. Medical terminology or abbreviations encountered:

____

____

6. Other observations:

____

____

Supervisor Signature: ______________________________

Date: ______________________________

Rotation Journal

Instructions: Write a journal entry detailing your learning experience at the clinical rotation. Use the following topics to help write a complete journal entry.

Assessment of the Environment

- Personnel
- Services provided
- Equipment
- Technology utilized

Observation

- Health care providers
- Team skills
- Communication skills
- Safety procedures
- Therapeutic/diagnostic procedures

Knowledge

- New information learned
- Medical terminology
- Skills learned

Evaluation

- Personal experience
- Educational value
- Professional value

Journal Entry

Write a journal entry summarizing your clinical experience.

____

____

____

____

____

____

Name ______ Date ______ Period ______

Health Informatics Pre-Clinical Worksheet

Instructions: Answer the following questions.

1. Define the following terms related to insurance.

A. Coinsurance:

______

______

B. Co-pay:

______

______

C. Deductible:

______

______

D. DRG:

______

______

E. EOB:

______

______

F. HMO:

______

______

G. Insurance fraud:

______

______

H. Out-of-pocket max:

______

______

I. PPO:

______

______

J. Premium:

______

______

(Continued)

K. Superbill:

L. Tickler report:

M. Worker's compensation:

2. How are Medicare and Medicaid alike? How are the two different?

3. In terms of insurance, who is the *beneficiary*, and who is the *insured*?

4. How do billing departments utilize collection agencies? Why might that not be in their best interest?

5. What does a medical coder do?

6. How is a certified administrative medical assistant different from a certified clinical medical assistant?

7. What types of tasks would an administrative medical assistant perform in a clinical office?

8. What types of personality traits do you feel would make an individual well suited for this career path?

9. What types of technical skills would be helpful for individuals pursuing this career path?

(Continued)

Name ____________________

10. Explain an administrative medical assistant's role in maintaining HIPAA.

11. What is the salary range for an administrative medical assistant?

12. Describe how you would answer the phone at the facility where you will attend clinical rotations.

13. If you have a disgruntled client approach you at the clinic, explain how you would handle it.

14. In what types of facilities might an administrative medical assistant work?

15. What type of education or certification is required to become an administrative medical assistant?

16. What are health informatics?

17. What career paths are included in the health informatics pathway?

18. What are some benefits of health informatics?

19. What are some HIPAA concerns related to electronic health records?

20. How would you protect private client information?

21. How do you think advances in technology have affected healthcare?

(Continued)

22. Why would knowledge of medical terminology be important in the field of health informatics?

____

____

23. Why is accuracy important when dealing with client records?

____

____

24. What is the Center for Medicaid and Medicare Services?

____

____

25. What is compliance? How would that relate to client information?

____

____

26. What would a medical chart auditor do?

____

____

27. What is the purpose of a chart audit?

____

____

Name ____________________ Date ____________ Period ____________

Health Informatics Workplace Discovery Sheet

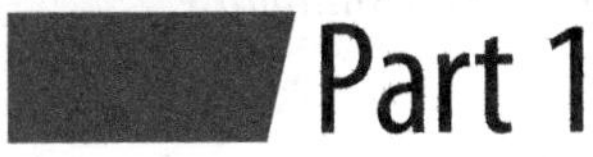

Part 1

During the Clinical Experience

Instructions: Answer the following questions.

1. What does a health informatics health care provider do?

____

____

2. What education and training are necessary to work in health informatics?

____

____

3. What equipment do you enjoy working with the most? Least?

____

____

4. What do you like most about this career?

____

____

5. What advice would you have for others who want to do similar work?

____

____

6. What additional courses do you wish you had taken in high school or college?

____

____

7. What is quality assurance?

____

____

8. What medical terms or abbreviations do you commonly use?

____

____

(Continued)

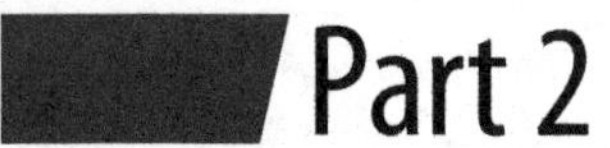 Part 2

After the Clinical Experience

Instructions: For each item below, identify whether you observed or assisted. Then, provide a brief summary.

Information Handling and Processing

1. Assembling records
   - ☐ Observed
   - ☐ Assisted

   Brief summary:

   ____

   ____

2. Accessing records
   - ☐ Observed
   - ☐ Assisted

   Brief summary:

   ____

   ____

3. Processing records
   - ☐ Observed
   - ☐ Assisted

   Brief summary:

   ____

   ____

4. Maintaining records
   - ☐ Observed
   - ☐ Assisted

   Brief summary:

   ____

   ____

5. Client's right to information
   - ☐ Observed
   - ☐ Assisted

   Brief summary:

   ____

   ____

(Continued)

Name ______________________________

6. Release of information
   - ☐ Observed
   - ☐ Assisted

   Brief summary:

   ____

   ____

7. Confidentiality
   - ☐ Observed
   - ☐ Assisted

   Brief summary:

   ____

   ____

8. Processing requests
   - ☐ Observed
   - ☐ Assisted

   Brief summary:

   ____

   ____

Technology Management

9. Software used
   - ☐ Observed
   - ☐ Assisted

   Brief summary:

   ____

   ____

10. Hardware used
    - ☐ Observed
    - ☐ Assisted

    Brief summary:

    ____

    ____

11. Staff access
    - ☐ Observed
    - ☐ Assisted

    Brief summary:

    ____

    ____

(Continued)

12. Ensuring accuracy
    ☐ Observed
    ☐ Assisted
    Brief summary:

    ____

    ____

13. Skills required
    ☐ Observed
    ☐ Assisted
    Brief summary:

    ____

    ____

Numbering and Filing Records

14. Organizational patterns
    ☐ Observed
    ☐ Assisted
    Brief summary:

    ____

    ____

15. Coding and indexing systems
    ☐ Observed
    ☐ Assisted
    Brief summary:

    ____

    ____

16. Other records/documents
    ☐ Observed
    ☐ Assisted
    Brief summary:

    ____

    ____

Client Records

17. Assembling charts
    ☐ Observed
    ☐ Assisted
    Brief summary:

    ____

    ____

(Continued)

Name ______________________________

18. Recording information
    ☐ Observed
    ☐ Assisted
    Brief summary:
    ____
    ____

19. Validating insurance
    ☐ Observed
    ☐ Assisted
    Brief summary:
    ____
    ____

20. Processing payments
    ☐ Observed
    ☐ Assisted
    Brief summary:
    ____
    ____

Office Management

21. Scheduling appointments
    ☐ Observed
    ☐ Assisted
    Brief summary:
    ____
    ____

22. Managing inventory
    ☐ Observed
    ☐ Assisted
    Brief summary:
    ____
    ____

23. Ordering supplies
    ☐ Observed
    ☐ Assisted
    Brief summary:
    ____
    ____

(Continued)

Procedures Special to this Office

24. Coding

    ☐ Observed

    ☐ Assisted

    Brief summary:

    ____

    ____

25. Filing claims

    ☐ Observed

    ☐ Assisted

    Brief summary:

    ____

    ____

Student Name: ________________________________

Technician Name: ______________________________

Student ______________________ Dates ____________ Site ____________ Preceptor ____________

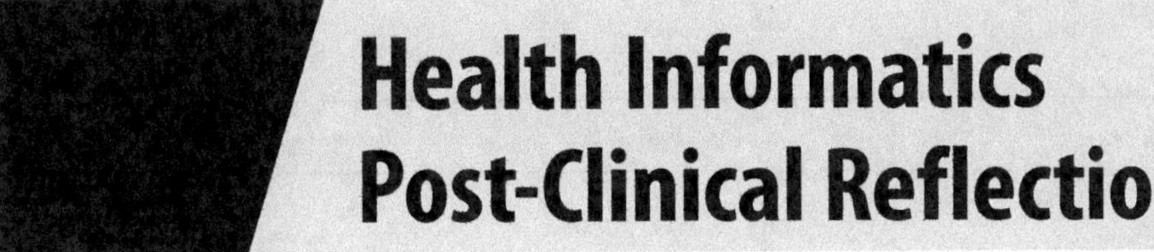

Health Informatics Post-Clinical Reflection

Rotation Report

Overview

Instructions: Answer the following questions using complete sentences.

1. What were your responsibilities or duties this week?

____

____

2. What new knowledge or skill did you learn or observe this week?

____

____

3. What was the best thing that happened at your clinical site this week?

____

____

4. What was the most challenging thing that happened at your clinical site this week?

____

____

5. What problems or difficulties did you encounter or observe at your clinical site? How were they dealt with?

____

____

6. Was this week good, fair, or bad? Explain.

____

____

Observations

Instructions: List the observations you made for each of the following categories.

1. Technology observed:

____

____

2. Diagnostic procedures observed:

____

____

(Continued)

3. Therapeutic procedures observed:

____

____

4. Diseases or disorders observed:

____

____

5. Medical terminology or abbreviations encountered:

____

____

6. Other observations:

____

____

Supervisor Signature: ____________________________

Date: ____________________________

Rotation Journal

Instructions: Write a journal entry detailing your learning experience at the clinical rotation. Use the following topics to help write a complete journal entry.

Assessment of the Environment

- Personnel
- Services provided
- Equipment
- Technology utilized

Observation

- Health care providers
- Team skills
- Communication skills
- Safety procedures
- Therapeutic/diagnostic procedures

Knowledge

- New information learned
- Medical terminology
- Skills learned

Evaluation

- Personal experience
- Educational value
- Professional value

Journal Entry

Write a journal entry summarizing your clinical experience.

____

____

____

____

____

____

Name ______________________ Date ______________ Period ____________

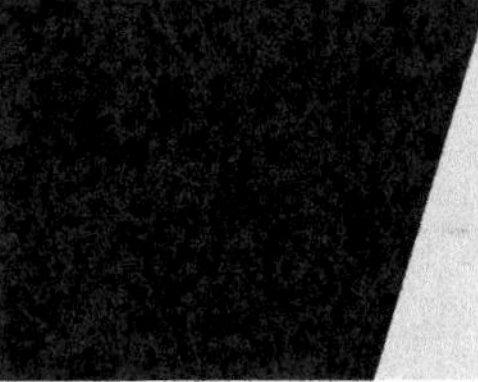

Laboratory Services Pre-Clinical Worksheet

Instructions: Answer the following questions.

1. Label the diagram of the major veins and arteries.

A. ______________________

B. ______________________

C. ______________________

D. ______________________

E. ______________________

F. ______________________

G. ______________________

H. ______________________

I. ______________________

J. ______________________

K. ______________________

L. ______________________

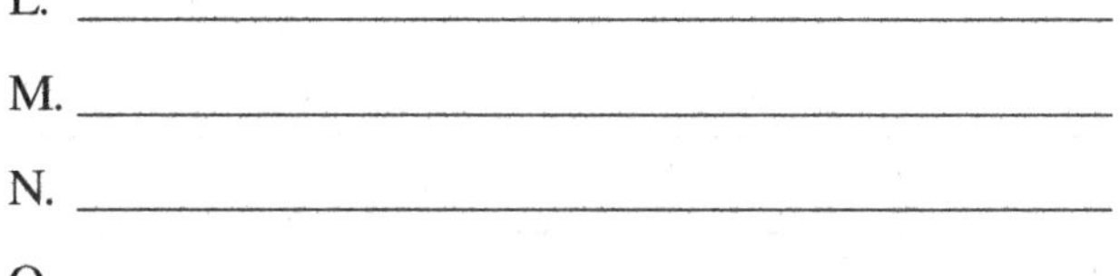

M. ______________________

N. ______________________

O. ______________________

P. ______________________

Q. ______________________

R. ______________________

S. ______________________

T. ______________________

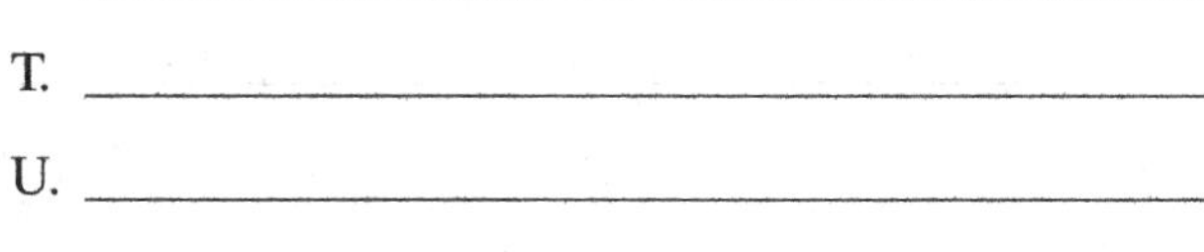

U. ______________________

V. ______________________

W. ______________________

X. ______________________

Y. ______________________

Z. ______________________

AA. ______________________

AB. ______________________

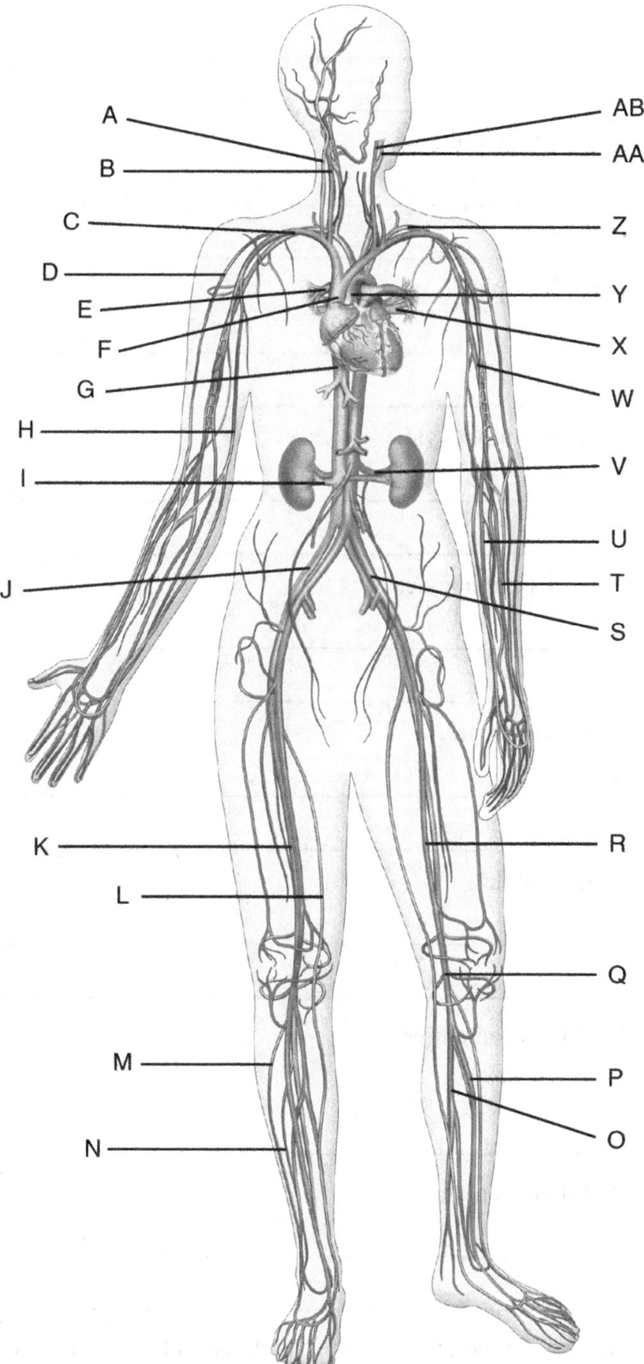

© Body Scientific International

(Continued)

2. Briefly describe the basic function of the following cells.

A. Red blood cell:

B. White blood cell:

C. Neutrophil:

D. Eosinophil:

E. Basophil:

F. B lymphocyte:

G. T lymphocyte:

H. Monocyte:

I. Platelet:

3. What is an antigen?

4. What is an antibody?

5. Explain the difference between natural and acquired immunity.

(Continued)

Name ____

6. Describe the blood types and their percentage found in the US population.

____

____

7. What is the Rh factor?

____

____

8. When collecting blood for testing, different colored tubes are used to indicate the type of additive being used. Research the following tube colors, then record their corresponding additive and what it does to the specimen.

   A. Lavender:

   ____

   B. Blue:

   ____

   C. Dark green:

   ____

   D. Red (plain):

   ____

   E. Red top with gel:

   ____

   F. Spotted:

   ____

   G. Yellow:

   ____

9. Define the following terms for classifying diseases and conditions, then provide an example of each.

   A. Acute:

   ____

   ____

   B. Autoimmune:

   ____

   ____

   C. Benign:

   ____

   ____

   D. Chronic:

   ____

   ____

   E. Congenital:

   ____

   ____

(Continued)

F. Debilitating:

G. Endemic:

H. Epidemic:

I. Genetic:

J. Hypersensitivity:

K. Iatrogenic:

L. Idiopathic:

M. Immunological:

N. Infectious:

O. Inflammatory:

P. Ischemic:

Q. Malignant:

(Continued)

Name ______________________________

R. Metabolic:

S. Neoplastic:

T. Nosocomial:

U. Nutritional:

V. Opportunistic:

W. Pandemic:

X. Terminal:

10. Explain the difference between a gross exam, frozen section exam, and microscopic exam.

11. If urine or blood toxicology is ordered, what are they looking for?

12. Interpret the following common lab abbreviations:

A. CBC:

B. RBC:

C. WBC:

D. Plt:

(Continued)

E. BUN/Creatinine: ______

F. Diff: ______

G. TNTC: ______

H. Hct: ______

I. Hgb: ______

J. Type and cross: ______

K. UA: ______

Name ______________________ Date ______________ Period ____________

Laboratory Services Workplace Discovery Sheet

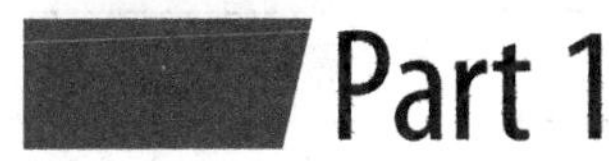

Part 1

During the Clinical Experience

Instructions: Answer the following questions.

1. What is the purpose of an anticoagulant?

2. Why is order of draw important?

3. What is the protocol for an accidental needle stick?

4. What is the most common stain used for tissues other than blood?

5. What is the most common stain used on blood?

6. What is the most common specimen sent to the lab for culture and sensitivity?

7. What are the different steps taken to grow an anaerobic culture?

8. Does the lab receive an order for a type and crossmatch for most surgery clients?

(Continued)

9. What is the most common serology test run at your facility? Does it change at different times of the year?

____

____

10. If the test is for something contagious, who is responsible for reporting the infection to the health department?

____

____

11. What is the most commonly ordered chemistry test in your facility?

____

____

Part 2

After the Clinical Experience

Instructions: For each item below, identify whether you observed or assisted. Then, provide a brief summary.

Safety

1. Infection control
   - ☐ Observed
   - ☐ Assisted

   Brief summary:

   ____

   ____

2. Fire safety
   - ☐ Observed
   - ☐ Assisted

   Brief summary:

   ____

   ____

Specimen Collection and Processing

3. Types of specimens
   - ☐ Observed
   - ☐ Assisted

   Brief summary:

   ____

   ____

(Continued)

Name ____

4. Supplies/equipment/techniques
   ☐ Observed
   ☐ Assisted
   Brief summary:
   ____
   ____

Hematology Procedures

5. Manual WBC, RBC, platelet count
   ☐ Observed
   ☐ Assisted
   Brief summary:
   ____
   ____

6. Blood smear preparation
   ☐ Observed
   ☐ Assisted
   Brief summary:
   ____
   ____

7. Cell ID and differentiation
   ☐ Observed
   ☐ Assisted
   Brief summary:
   ____
   ____

8. Coagulation studies
   ☐ Observed
   ☐ Assisted
   Brief summary:
   ____
   ____

Chemistry Procedures

9. Routine chemistry tests
   ☐ Observed
   ☐ Assisted
   Brief summary:
   ____
   ____

(Continued)

10. Drug assays
    ☐ Observed
    ☐ Assisted
    Brief summary:

    ____

    ____

11. Isoenzymes
    ☐ Observed
    ☐ Assisted
    Brief summary:

    ____

    ____

12. Immunoassays
    ☐ Observed
    ☐ Assisted
    Brief summary:

    ____

    ____

13. Electrophoresis
    ☐ Observed
    ☐ Assisted
    Brief summary:

    ____

    ____

Blood Bank

14. ABO and Rh blood group systems
    ☐ Observed
    ☐ Assisted
    Brief summary:

    ____

    ____

15. Antiglobulin testing
    ☐ Observed
    ☐ Assisted
    Brief summary:

    ____

    ____

(Continued)

Name ____________________________

16. Compatibility testing
    ☐ Observed
    ☐ Assisted
    Brief summary:

    ____

    ____

17. Hemolytic diseases
    ☐ Observed
    ☐ Assisted
    Brief summary:

    ____

    ____

18. Blood preparation/storage
    ☐ Observed
    ☐ Assisted
    Brief summary:

    ____

    ____

Microbiology

19. Culture inoculation
    ☐ Observed
    ☐ Assisted
    Brief summary:

    ____

    ____

20. Gram stain preparation/procedure
    ☐ Observed
    ☐ Assisted
    Brief summary:

    ____

    ____

21. Culture interpretation
    ☐ Observed
    ☐ Assisted
    Brief summary:

    ____

    ____

(Continued)

22. Organism ID and antibiotic sensitivity
    ☐ Observed
    ☐ Assisted
    Brief summary:

Urinalysis and Serology Procedures

23. Chemical analysis
    ☐ Observed
    ☐ Assisted
    Brief summary:

24. Microscopic exam of sediment
    ☐ Observed
    ☐ Assisted
    Brief summary:

25. Qualitative serological tests
    ☐ Observed
    ☐ Assisted
    Brief summary:

Histology Procedures

26. Gross exam
    ☐ Observed
    ☐ Assisted
    Brief summary:

27. Processing/embedding/cutting specimens
    ☐ Observed
    ☐ Assisted
    Brief summary:

(Continued)

Name ______________________________

28. Staining slides
    - ☐ Observed
    - ☐ Assisted

    Brief summary:

    ____

    ____

Phlebotomy Skills

29. Client identification
    - ☐ Observed
    - ☐ Assisted

    Brief summary:

    ____

    ____

30. Finding the right vein
    - ☐ Observed
    - ☐ Assisted

    Brief summary:

    ____

    ____

31. Order of draw
    - ☐ Observed
    - ☐ Assisted

    Brief summary:

    ____

    ____

32. Collection procedure
    - ☐ Observed
    - ☐ Assisted

    Brief summary:

    ____

    ____

Student Name: ______________________________

Technician Name: ______________________________

Notes

Student ______________________ Dates ____________ Site ____________ Preceptor ____________

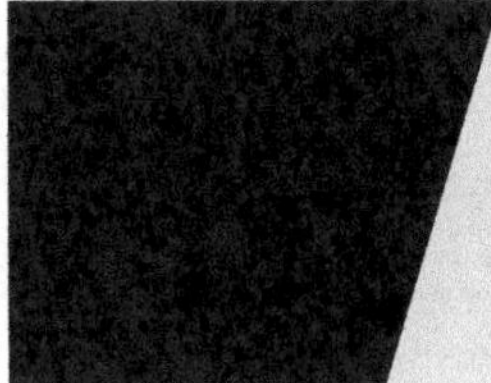

Laboratory Services Post-Clinical Reflection

Rotation Report

Overview

Instructions: Answer the following questions using complete sentences.

1. What were your responsibilities or duties this week?

____

____

2. What new knowledge or skill did you learn or observe this week?

____

____

3. What was the best thing that happened at your clinical site this week?

____

____

4. What was the most challenging thing that happened at your clinical site this week?

____

____

5. What problems or difficulties did you encounter or observe at your clinical site? How were they dealt with?

____

____

6. Was this week good, fair, or bad? Explain.

____

____

Observations

Instructions: List the observations you made for each of the following categories.

1. Technology observed:

____

____

2. Diagnostic procedures observed:

____

____

(Continued)

3. Therapeutic procedures observed:

____

____

4. Diseases or disorders observed:

____

____

5. Medical terminology or abbreviations encountered:

____

____

6. Other observations:

____

____

Student Name: ______________________________

Technicians Name: ______________________________

Rotation Journal

Instructions: Write a journal entry detailing your learning experience at the clinical rotation. Use the following topics to help write a complete journal entry.

Assessment of the Environment

- Personnel
- Services provided
- Equipment
- Technology utilized

Observation

- Health care providers
- Team skills
- Communication skills
- Safety procedures
- Therapeutic/diagnostic procedures

Knowledge

- New information learned
- Medical terminology
- Skills learned

Evaluation

- Personal experience
- Educational value
- Professional value

Journal Entry

Write a journal entry summarizing your clinical experience.

____

____

____

____

____

____

Name ______________________ Date ____________ Period ____________

Mortuary Services Pre-Clinical Worksheet

Instructions: Answer the following questions.

1. Why is it important for funeral service professionals to develop relationships with the families and communities they serve?

2. How is a funeral different from a memorial service?

3. What is a eulogy?

4. What are the basic costs for traditional burial versus cremation?

5. Do cemeteries usually require grave liners or urn vaults?

6. How is a living will different from a standard will?

7. What types of clients may require special adjustments or may be difficult to adjust?

8. What kind of duties would a funeral director have?

9. Do you have to go to college to become a funeral director?

(Continued)

10. Why do you think a funeral director would need to have strong communication skills?

____

____

11. Define the following terms related to mortuary services.

A. Embalming:

____

____

B. Visitation:

____

____

C. Death certificate:

____

____

D. Cremation:

____

____

E. Human remains:

____

____

F. Obituary:

____

____

Name ____________________ Date ____________ Period __________

Mortuary Services Workplace Discovery Sheet

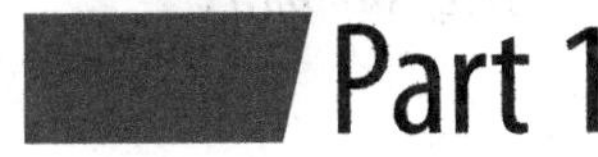

Part 1

During the Clinical Experience

Instructions: Answer the following questions.

1. What does a mortuary services provider do?

____

____

2. What education and training are necessary to work in mortuary services?

____

____

3. What do you like most about this career?

____

____

4. What advice would you have for others who want to do similar work?

____

____

5. What additional courses do you wish you had taken in high school or college?

____

____

6. What is quality assurance?

____

____

7. What medical terms or abbreviations do you commonly use?

____

____

(Continued)

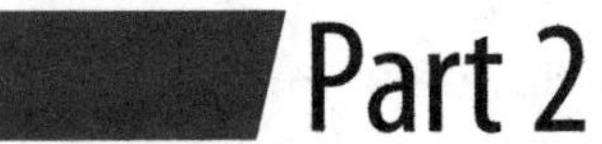

Part 2

After the Clinical Experience

Instructions: For each item below, identify whether you observed or assisted. Then, provide a brief summary.

Client Services

1. Visitation
   - ☐ Observed
   - ☐ Assisted

   Brief summary:

   ____

   ____

2. Funerals
   - ☐ Observed
   - ☐ Assisted

   Brief summary:

   ____

   ____

3. Cremation
   - ☐ Observed
   - ☐ Assisted

   Brief summary:

   ____

   ____

4. Memorial services
   - ☐ Observed
   - ☐ Assisted

   Brief summary:

   ____

   ____

5. Embalming
   - ☐ Observed
   - ☐ Assisted

   Brief summary:

   ____

   ____

(Continued)

Name ____

Career Path

6. Job duties
   - ☐ Observed
   - ☐ Assisted

   Brief summary:

   ____

   ____

7. Education
   - ☐ Observed
   - ☐ Assisted

   Brief summary:

   ____

   ____

8. Job growth
   - ☐ Observed
   - ☐ Assisted

   Brief summary:

   ____

   ____

Documentation

9. Licenses
   - ☐ Observed
   - ☐ Assisted

   Brief summary:

   ____

   ____

10. Death certificate
    - ☐ Observed
    - ☐ Assisted

    Brief summary:

    ____

    ____

11. Other legal documents
    - ☐ Observed
    - ☐ Assisted

    Brief summary:

    ____

    ____

(Continued)

Communication

12. Oral
    - ☐ Observed
    - ☐ Assisted

    Brief summary:

    ____

    ____

13. Written
    - ☐ Observed
    - ☐ Assisted

    Brief summary:

    ____

    ____

14. Electronic
    - ☐ Observed
    - ☐ Assisted

    Brief summary:

    ____

    ____

Resources

15. Support groups
    - ☐ Observed
    - ☐ Assisted

    Brief summary:

    ____

    ____

Student Name: ______________________________

Technician Name: ______________________________

Student ______________________ Dates ____________ Site ____________ Preceptor ____________

Mortuary Services Post-Clinical Reflection

Rotation Report

Overview

Instructions: Answer the following questions using complete sentences.

1. What were your responsibilities or duties this week?

____

____

2. What new knowledge or skill did you learn or observe this week?

____

____

3. What was the best thing that happened at your clinical site this week?

____

____

4. What was the most challenging thing that happened at your clinical site this week?

____

____

5. What problems or difficulties did you encounter or observe at your clinical site? How were they dealt with?

____

____

6. Was this week good, fair, or bad? Explain.

____

____

Observations

Instructions: List the observations you made for each of the following categories.

1. Technology observed:

____

____

2. Diagnostic procedures observed:

____

____

(Continued)

3. Therapeutic procedures observed:

____

____

4. Diseases or disorders observed:

____

____

5. Medical terminology or abbreviations encountered:

____

____

6. Other observations:

____

____

Supervisor Signature: ______________________________

Date: ______________________________

Rotation Journal

Instructions: Write a journal entry detailing your learning experience at the clinical rotation. Use the following topics to help write a complete journal entry.

Assessment of the Environment

- Personnel
- Services provided
- Equipment
- Technology utilized

Observation

- Health care providers
- Team skills
- Communication skills
- Safety procedures
- Therapeutic/diagnostic procedures

Knowledge

- New information learned
- Medical terminology
- Skills learned

Evaluation

- Personal experience
- Educational value
- Professional value

Journal Entry

Write a journal entry summarizing your clinical experience.

____

____

____

____

____

____

Name ________________ Date ________ Period ________

Nursing Pre-Clinical Worksheet

Instructions: Answer the following questions.

1. Where does the O_2/CO_2 exchange occur between the heart and the lungs?

2. Differentiate between an endotracheal tube and a tracheostomy tube.

3. What is enteral nutrition?

4. What are the signs and symptoms of respiratory failure?

5. What are the signs and symptoms of shock?

6. A basic neurological evaluation includes the following assessments. Briefly describe what happens in each step.
   A. Level of consciousness using the Glasgow Coma Scale:

   B. Pupillary response:

   C. Limb movement/strength:

   D. Vital signs:

(Continued)

7. In addition to medications and a defibrillator, the following items are commonly found on a crash cart. Briefly describe how each item is used.
   A. IV equipment:

   ____

   B. Suction supplies:

   ____

   C. Endotracheal tube:

   ____

   D. Laryngoscope:

   ____

   E. Bag valve mask:

   ____

   F. Magill forceps:

   ____

   G. Cricothyroidotomy kit:

   ____

8. Describe the methods for taking a client's temperature including the normal ranges.

____

9. What is the normal pulse range for an adult?

____

10. What is the level of blood pressure called when the heart muscle relaxes?

____

11. What is a normal range for an adult's blood pressure? What is the medical term for high blood pressure? What is the medical term for low blood pressure?

____

12. What does an abnormally low systolic blood pressure possibly indicate?

____

(Continued)

Name ____

13. List five factors that affect blood pressure.

____

____

14. What is the normal range for adult respirations?

____

15. Describe the following terms related to breathing.

A. Rales:

____

____

B. Diaphoretic:

____

____

C. Dyspnea:

____

____

D. Apnea:

____

____

E. Cheyne-Stokes:

____

____

16. Define the following terms associated with intake and output.

A. Dehydration:

____

____

B. Edema:

____

____

C. TPN:

____

____

D. Foley catheter:

____

____

(Continued)

E. Hemovac:

F. BM:

G. IV's:

H. Blood products:

I. Gavage:

J. Lavage:

K. Emesis:

L. Urine:

17. Define the following med terms.
    A. Anuria:

    B. Diuresis:

    C. Dysuria:

    D. Glycosuria:

(Continued)

Name ______________________________

E. Hematuria:

____

____

F. Oliguria:

____

____

G. Polyuria:

____

____

H. Urinary incontinence:

____

____

I. Urinary retention:

____

____

18. Interpret the following abbreviations.

A. AC:

____

B. BID:

____

C. BM:

____

D. BP:

____

E. CXR:

____

F. EKG:

____

G. HS:

____

H. I&O:

____

I. PC:

____

J. TID:

____

(Continued)

K. TPR:

____

L. Q4hr:

____

M. QID:

____

N. VS:

____

Name ______________________ Date ____________ Period ____________

Nursing Workplace Discovery Sheet

Part 1

During the Clinical Experience

Instructions: Answer the following questions.

1. Explain why a client is admitted to a critical care unit.

2. What is the average client/nurse ratio in your ICU/CCU?

3. Do you work mostly with the client's actual physician or the hospitalist?

4. How often do you reassess your clients coming from surgery?

5. What training/experience did you have before coming into the ICU/CCU?

6. What is a peripherally inserted central line used for? An arterial line?

7. What are the pros and the cons of parenteral and enteral nutrition?

8. Are all clients in ICU/CCU hooked up to telemetry?

(Continued)

9. When clients need specialized testing such as an MRI or CT scan, do you go with the client?

10. What is EEG used for?

11. What happens when all the rooms in ICU/CCU are full, and another client becomes critical?

12. Describe the purpose and procedure for helping a client dangle.

13. What PPE is required for each type of isolation (contact, airborne, droplet, and protective)?

14. What is the purpose of reverse isolation?

15. How often should clients be turned?

16. What type of clients are at increased risk for falls (list at least four reasons):

17. What type of interventions have been put in place to help prevent clients from falling on this unit? (List three or more.)

18. Which jobs on the unit are typically performed by the PCT/CAN? By the LVN? By the RN?

(Continued)

Name ____

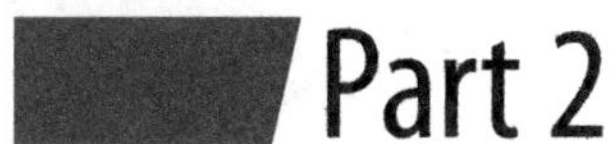

Part 2

After the Clinical Experience

Instructions: For each item below, identify whether you observed or assisted. Then, provide a brief summary.

Client Assessment

1. Standard precautions
   - ☐ Observed
   - ☐ Assisted

   Brief summary:

   ____

   ____

2. Client assessment
   - ☐ Observed
   - ☐ Assisted

   Brief summary:

   ____

   ____

3. Assessment of heart sounds
   - ☐ Observed
   - ☐ Assisted

   Brief summary:

   ____

   ____

4. Assessment of breath sounds
   - ☐ Observed
   - ☐ Assisted

   Brief summary:

   ____

   ____

Client Care

5. Admission procedures
   - ☐ Observed
   - ☐ Assisted

   Brief summary:

   ____

   ____

(Continued)

6. Discharge/Transfer procedures
   ☐ Observed
   ☐ Assisted
   Brief summary:

   ____

   ____

7. Skin care
   ☐ Observed
   ☐ Assisted
   Brief summary:

   ____

   ____

8. Tracheostomy care
   ☐ Observed
   ☐ Assisted
   Brief summary:

   ____

   ____

9. Endotracheal tube
   ☐ Observed
   ☐ Assisted
   Brief summary:

   ____

   ____

Equipment

10. EKG/Cardiac monitoring
    ☐ Observed
    ☐ Assisted
    Brief summary:

    ____

    ____

11. IV Infusion pump
    ☐ Observed
    ☐ Assisted
    Brief summary:

    ____

    ____

(Continued)

Name ____

12. Ventilators
    - ☐ Observed
    - ☐ Assisted

    Brief summary:

    ____

    ____

Infusion Lines

13. CVP millilumen catheter
    - ☐ Observed
    - ☐ Assisted

    Brief summary:

    ____

    ____

14. Arterial lines
    - ☐ Observed
    - ☐ Assisted

    Brief summary:

    ____

    ____

15. Thermodilution catheters
    - ☐ Observed
    - ☐ Assisted

    Brief summary:

    ____

    ____

Emergency Treatment

16. Arrhythmia client
    - ☐ Observed
    - ☐ Assisted

    Brief summary:

    ____

    ____

17. Bradycardia client
    - ☐ Observed
    - ☐ Assisted

    Brief summary:

    ____

    ____

(Continued)

18. Tachycardia client
    ☐ Observed
    ☐ Assisted
    Brief summary:

    ____

    ____

19. Cardiac arrest
    ☐ Observed
    ☐ Assisted
    Brief summary:

    ____

    ____

20. Defibrillation
    ☐ Observed
    ☐ Assisted
    Brief summary:

    ____

    ____

Safety Procedures

21. Emergency exits/fire extinguishers
    ☐ Observed
    ☐ Assisted
    Brief summary:

    ____

    ____

22. Crash cart/CPR
    ☐ Observed
    ☐ Assisted
    Brief summary:

    ____

    ____

23. Disaster procedures
    ☐ Observed
    ☐ Assisted
    Brief summary:

    ____

    ____

(Continued)

Name ______________________________

Infection Control

24. Universal precautions
    - ☐ Observed
    - ☐ Assisted

    Brief summary:

    ____

    ____

25. Isolation techniques
    - ☐ Observed
    - ☐ Assisted

    Brief summary:

    ____

    ____

AM Care

26. Bathing/Dressing clients
    - ☐ Observed
    - ☐ Assisted

    Brief summary:

    ____

    ____

27. Nourishments/Meals
    - ☐ Observed
    - ☐ Assisted

    Brief summary:

    ____

    ____

28. Changing bed linens
    - ☐ Observed
    - ☐ Assisted

    Brief summary:

    ____

    ____

29. Intake and output
    - ☐ Observed
    - ☐ Assisted

    Brief summary:

    ____

    ____

(Continued)

Wound Care

30. Dressing change
    ☐ Observed
    ☐ Assisted
    Brief summary:

    ____

    ____

31. Operative site check
    ☐ Observed
    ☐ Assisted
    Brief summary:

    ____

    ____

32. Suture removal
    ☐ Observed
    ☐ Assisted
    Brief summary:

    ____

    ____

Skills

33. Vital signs
    ☐ Observed
    ☐ Assisted
    Brief summary:

    ____

    ____

34. Ambulation
    ☐ Observed
    ☐ Assisted
    Brief summary:

    ____

    ____

35. Transporting clients
    ☐ Observed
    ☐ Assisted
    Brief summary:

    ____

    ____

(Continued)

36. Passing out medications

    ☐ Observed

    ☐ Assisted

    Brief summary:

    ____

    ____

37. Other assessments

    ☐ Observed

    ☐ Assisted

    Brief summary:

    ____

    ____

Student Name: ______________________________

Technician Name: ______________________________

Notes

Student ____________ Dates ____________ Site ____________ Preceptor ____________

Nursing Post-Clinical Reflection

Rotation Report

Overview

Instructions: Answer the following questions using complete sentences.

1. What were your responsibilities or duties this week?

2. What new knowledge or skill did you learn or observe this week?

3. What was the best thing that happened at your clinical site this week?

4. What was the most challenging thing that happened at your clinical site this week?

5. What problems or difficulties did you encounter or observe at your clinical site? How were they dealt with?

6. Was this week good, fair, or bad? Explain.

Observations

Instructions: List the observations you made for each of the following categories.

1. Technology observed:

2. Diagnostic procedures observed:

(Continued)

3. Therapeutic procedures observed:

____

____

4. Diseases or disorders observed:

____

____

5. Medical terminology or abbreviations encountered:

____

____

6. Other observations:

____

____

Supervisor Signature: ______________________

Date: ______________________

Rotation Journal

Instructions: Write a journal entry detailing your learning experience at the clinical rotation. Use the following topics to help write a complete journal entry.

Assessment of the Environment

- Personnel
- Services provided
- Equipment
- Technology utilized

Observation

- Health care providers
- Team skills
- Communication skills
- Safety procedures
- Therapeutic/diagnostic procedures

Knowledge

- New information learned
- Medical terminology
- Skills learned

Evaluation

- Personal experience
- Educational value
- Professional value

Journal Entry

Write a journal entry summarizing your clinical experience.

____

____

____

____

____

____

Name ______________________ Date __________ Period __________

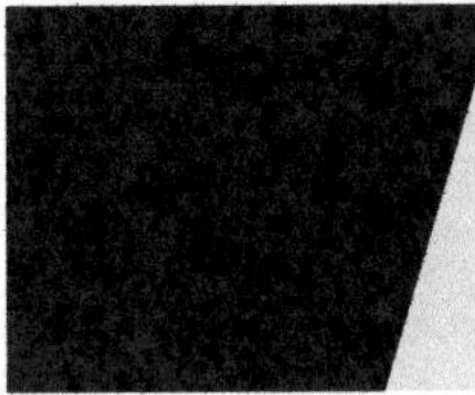

Oncology Pre-Clinical Worksheet

Instructions: Answer the following questions.

1. Define the following terms.

A. Acute:

____

____

B. Benign:

____

____

C. Cancer:

____

____

D. Chronic:

____

____

E. Genetic:

____

____

F. Iatrogenic:

____

____

G. Idiopathic:

____

____

H. Malignant:

____

____

I. Metastasis:

____

____

J. Neoplastic:

____

____

(Continued)

K. Opportunistic:

L. Prophylaxis:

M. Remission:

N. Staging:

O. Terminal:

2. Define the following types of treatments for cancer.
   A. Chemotherapy:

   B. Radiation therapy:

   C. Immunotherapy:

   D. Surgery:

   E. Bone marrow transplant

3. Research the following common types of cancer, then record their types, signs and symptoms, etiology, preventions, treatments, and prognoses.
   A. Skin:

(Continued)

Name ______________________________

B. Leukemia

____

____

____

C. Lung:

____

____

____

D. Colon:

____

____

____

E. Breast:

____

____

____

F. Prostate:

____

____

____

G. Lymphoma:

____

____

____

Notes

Name ______________________ Date ____________ Period ____________

Oncology Workplace Discovery Sheet

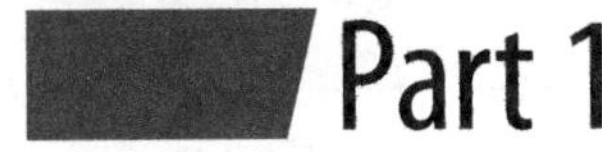

Part 1

During the Clinical Experience

Instructions: Answer the following questions.

1. What client/staff safety measures are utilized with radiation therapy?

2. How does radiation therapy work?

3. How long does an individual treatment take?

4. What are the common side effects of radiation therapy?

5. How long will most cancers require radiation therapy?

6. What client/staff safety measures are utilized with chemotherapy treatments?

7. How does chemotherapy work?

8. What are the common side effects of chemotherapy?

(Continued)

9. How long does it normally take to infuse chemotherapy?

____

____

10. What types of blood tests are usually ordered or monitored on clients receiving chemotherapy?

____

____

11. Chemotherapies given intravenously frequently cause damage to the vein. Often physicians will surgically implant a chemo port. Compare and contrast peripheral IV lines, PICC ports, and CVC ports.

____

____

____

12. What type of cancers are treated with oral chemotherapy?

____

____

13. What are the most common opportunist infections cancer clients get?

____

____

14. Do most clients still receive either chemo or radiation therapy after surgery to remove a tumor? What does the usual follow-up treatment look like?

____

____

15. What types of cancers are treated by a bone marrow transplant?

____

____

Part 2

After the Clinical Experience

Instructions: For each item below, identify whether you observed or assisted. Then, provide a brief summary.

Basic Client Care

1. Assessment/Vital signs
   ☐ Observed
   ☐ Assisted
   Brief summary:

____

____

(Continued)

Name ______________________________

2. Height and weight measurement
   - ☐ Observed
   - ☐ Assisted

   Brief summary:

   ____

   ____

3. Intake and output
   - ☐ Observed
   - ☐ Assisted

   Brief summary:

   ____

   ____

4. Bathing and AM care
   - ☐ Observed
   - ☐ Assisted

   Brief summary:

   ____

   ____

5. Moving, lifting, positioning
   - ☐ Observed
   - ☐ Assisted

   Brief summary:

   ____

   ____

6. Nourishment/Meals
   - ☐ Observed
   - ☐ Assisted

   Brief summary:

   ____

   ____

Universal Precautions

7. Isolation
   - ☐ Observed
   - ☐ Assisted

   Brief summary:

   ____

   ____

(Continued)

8. Reverse isolation
   ☐ Observed
   ☐ Assisted
   Brief summary:

Special Procedures

9. Chemotherapy
   ☐ Observed
   ☐ Assisted
   Brief summary:

10. Thoracentesis/Paracentesis
    ☐ Observed
    ☐ Assisted
    Brief summary:

11. Hyperalimentation
    ☐ Observed
    ☐ Assisted
    Brief summary:

12. Biopsy
    ☐ Observed
    ☐ Assisted
    Brief summary:

13. Bone marrow aspiration
    ☐ Observed
    ☐ Assisted
    Brief summary:

(Continued)

Name ____________________

The Terminal Client

14. Stages of grief
    - ☐ Observed
    - ☐ Assisted

    Brief summary:

    ____

    ____

15. Psychological needs of client/family
    - ☐ Observed
    - ☐ Assisted

    Brief summary:

    ____

    ____

16. Hospice care
    - ☐ Observed
    - ☐ Assisted

    Brief summary:

    ____

    ____

17. Advanced directives
    - ☐ Observed
    - ☐ Assisted

    Brief summary:

    ____

    ____

18. DNR/No Code
    - ☐ Observed
    - ☐ Assisted

    Brief summary:

    ____

    ____

19. Signs of approaching death
    - ☐ Observed
    - ☐ Assisted

    Brief summary:

    ____

    ____

(Continued)

20. Care of the deceased

☐ Observed

☐ Assisted

Brief summary:

____

____

21. Death certificate

☐ Observed

☐ Assisted

Brief summary:

____

____

Student Name: ______________________________

Technician Name: ____________________________

Student ______________________ Dates __________ Site __________ Preceptor __________

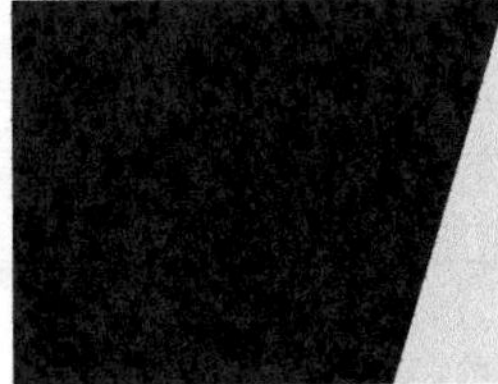

Oncology Post-Clinical Reflection

Rotation Report

Overview

Instructions: Answer the following questions using complete sentences.

1. What were your responsibilities or duties this week?

2. What new knowledge or skill did you learn or observe this week?

3. What was the best thing that happened at your clinical site this week?

4. What was the most challenging thing that happened at your clinical site this week?

5. What problems or difficulties did you encounter or observe at your clinical site? How were they dealt with?

6. Was this week good, fair, or bad? Explain.

Observations

Instructions: List the observations you made for each of the following categories.

1. Technology observed:

2. Diagnostic procedures observed:

(Continued)

3. Therapeutic procedures observed:

____

____

4. Diseases or disorders observed:

____

____

5. Medical terminology or abbreviations encountered:

____

____

6. Other observations:

____

____

Supervisor Signature: ______________________________

Date: ______________________________

Rotation Journal

Instructions: Write a journal entry detailing your learning experience at the clinical rotation. Use the following topics to help write a complete journal entry.

Assessment of the Environment

- Personnel
- Services provided
- Equipment
- Technology utilized

Observation

- Health care providers
- Team skills
- Communication skills
- Safety procedures
- Therapeutic/diagnostic procedures

Knowledge

- New information learned
- Medical terminology
- Skills learned

Evaluation

- Personal experience
- Educational value
- Professional value

Journal Entry

Write a journal entry summarizing your clinical experience.

____

____

____

____

____

____

Name ______________________ Date ____________ Period ________

Optical Pre-Clinical Worksheet

Instructions: Answer the following questions.

1. What is the difference between an optician, an optometrist, and an ophthalmologist?

____

____

2. Label the following diagram of the eye.

A. ______________________

B. ______________________

C. ______________________

D. ______________________

E. ______________________

F. ______________________

G. ______________________

H. ______________________

I. ______________________

J. ______________________

K. ______________________

L. ______________________

M. ______________________

N. ______________________

O. ______________________

© *Body Scientific International*

3. Describe the primary function of the following parts of the eye.

A. Conjunctiva:

____

____

B. Sclera:

____

____

C. Cornea:

____

____

(Continued)

D. Pupil:

E. Lens:

F. Iris:

G. Optic nerve:

H. Retina:

I. Aqueous humor:

J. Rods:

K. Cones:

L. Lacrimal glands:

4. Define the following eye conditions.
   A. Amblyopia:

   B. Blepharitis:

   C. Cataract:

(Continued)

Name ______________________________

D. Chalazion:

____

____

E. Dacryocystitis:

____

____

F. Diabetic retinopathy:

____

____

G. Glaucoma:

____

____

H. Hordeolum:

____

____

I. Macular degeneration:

____

____

J. Nystagmus:

____

____

K. Astigmatism:

____

____

L. Hyperopia:

____

____

M. Myopia:

____

____

N. Presbyopia:

____

____

O. Retinal detachment:

____

____

(Continued)

P. Strabismus:

5. Define the following procedures pertaining to the eye.
   A. Fluorescein angiography:

   B. Ishihara color vision:

   C. Keratometry:

   D. Ophthalmoscopy:

   E. Slit lamp microscopy:

   F. Visual acuity test:

   G. Visual field test:

6. Describe the following types of eye surgery.
   A. Vision correction (LASIK and PRK):

   B. Cataract surgery:

   C. Corneal transplant:

(Continued)

Name ______________________________

D. Strabismus surgery:

____

____

E. Surgery to repair an open globe injury:

____

____

F. Surgery for glaucoma:

____

____

G. Enucleation:

____

____

Notes

Name ______________________ Date ____________ Period ____________

Optical Workplace Discovery Sheet

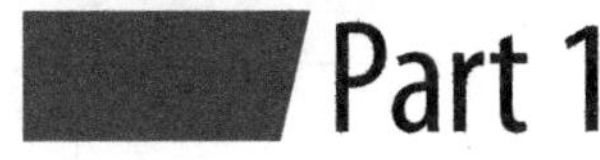

Part 1

During the Clinical Experience

Instructions: Answer the following questions.

1. What type of tests are performed in this office?

2. Are there designated stations or rooms for different procedures? Do they have specific names?

3. How many different types of eye care professionals are there? What type of training is required for each?

4. What are the typical vision problems seen in this office and how they are treated?

5. What type/classification of medications are used for the eye?

6. What does 20/20 mean? What does 20/1000 mean?

7. Give the meaning of the following abbreviations.
   A. ARMD:

   B. BID:

   C. CE:

(Continued)

D. CS:

E. LASIK:

F. NPDR:

G. OD:

H. OS:

I. OU:

J. PERRLA/PERRL/PEAR:

K. QID:

L. RX:

M. TID:

Part 2

After the Clinical Experience

Instructions: For each item below, identify whether you observed or assisted. Then, provide a brief summary.

Administrative

1. Charting
   - ☐ Observed
   - ☐ Assisted

   Brief summary:

(Continued)

Name ______________________________

2. Computer record keeping
   - ☐ Observed
   - ☐ Assisted

   Brief summary:

   ____

   ____

3. Checking patients in and out
   - ☐ Observed
   - ☐ Assisted

   Brief summary:

   ____

   ____

Assessment

4. Glaucoma exam
   - ☐ Observed
   - ☐ Assisted

   Brief summary:

   ____

   ____

5. Vision exam
   - ☐ Observed
   - ☐ Assisted

   Brief summary:

   ____

   ____

6. Cataract exam
   - ☐ Observed
   - ☐ Assisted

   Brief summary:

   ____

   ____

7. Eye pressure exam
   - ☐ Observed
   - ☐ Assisted

   Brief summary:

   ____

   ____

(Continued)

8. Vision field test–Humphrey/Goldman
   - ☐ Observed
   - ☐ Assisted

   Brief summary:

   ____

   ____

9. Slit lamp exam
   - ☐ Observed
   - ☐ Assisted

   Brief summary:

   ____

   ____

10. External exam
    - ☐ Observed
    - ☐ Assisted

    Brief summary:

    ____

    ____

11. Refractions
    - ☐ Observed
    - ☐ Assisted

    Brief summary:

    ____

    ____

12. Complete eye exam
    - ☐ Observed
    - ☐ Assisted

    Brief summary:

    ____

    ____

13. Fundus exam
    - ☐ Observed
    - ☐ Assisted

    Brief summary:

    ____

    ____

(Continued)

Name ______________________________

Equipment

14. Lensometer

☐ Observed

☐ Assisted

Brief summary:

____

____

15. Snellen Chart

☐ Observed

☐ Assisted

Brief summary:

____

____

16. Ophthalmoscope–direct/indirect

☐ Observed

☐ Assisted

Brief summary:

____

____

17. Slit lamp

☐ Observed

☐ Assisted

Brief summary:

____

____

18. Tonometer

☐ Observed

☐ Assisted

Brief summary:

____

____

19. Retinoscope

☐ Observed

☐ Assisted

Brief summary:

____

____

(Continued)

20. Potential Acuity Meter (PAM)
   ☐ Observed
   ☐ Assisted
   Brief summary:

   ____

   ____

Other

21. Lens terms and classification
   ☐ Observed
   ☐ Assisted
   Brief summary:

   ____

   ____

22. Light and light refraction
   ☐ Observed
   ☐ Assisted
   Brief summary:

   ____

   ____

23. Using measuring instruments
   ☐ Observed
   ☐ Assisted
   Brief summary:

   ____

   ____

24. Lens prescriptions and calculations
   ☐ Observed
   ☐ Assisted
   Brief summary:

   ____

   ____

25. Lens production
   ☐ Observed
   ☐ Assisted
   Brief summary:

   ____

   ____

(Continued)

Name ____________________

26. Eyeglass assembly, alignment, quality control
    - ☐ Observed
    - ☐ Assisted

    Brief summary:

    ____

    ____

27. Owning an optical business
    - ☐ Observed
    - ☐ Assisted

    Brief summary:

    ____

    ____

28. Eye functions and deficiencies
    - ☐ Observed
    - ☐ Assisted

    Brief summary:

    ____

    ____

29. Human relations in business ownership
    - ☐ Observed
    - ☐ Assisted

    Brief summary:

    ____

    ____

Student Name: ____________________

Technician Name: ____________________

Notes

Student ______________________ Dates __________ Site __________ Preceptor __________

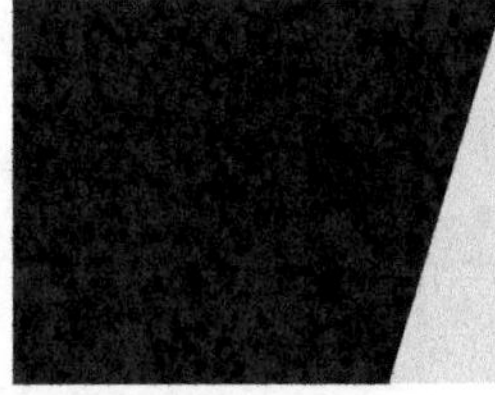

Optical Post-Clinical Reflection

Rotation Report

Overview

Instructions: Answer the following questions using complete sentences.

1. What were your responsibilities or duties this week?

____

____

2. What new knowledge or skill did you learn or observe this week?

____

____

3. What was the best thing that happened at your clinical site this week?

____

____

4. What was the most challenging thing that happened at your clinical site this week?

____

____

5. What problems or difficulties did you encounter or observe at your clinical site? How were they dealt with?

____

____

6. Was this week good, fair, or bad? Explain.

____

____

Observations

Instructions: List the observations you made for each of the following categories.

1. Technology observed:

____

____

2. Diagnostic procedures observed:

____

____

(Continued)

3. Therapeutic procedures observed:

____

____

4. Diseases or disorders observed:

____

____

5. Medical terminology or abbreviations encountered:

____

____

6. Other observations:

____

____

Supervisor Signature: ______________________________

Date: ______________________________

Rotation Journal

Instructions: Write a journal entry detailing your learning experience at the clinical rotation. Use the following topics to help write a complete journal entry.

Assessment of the Environment

- Personnel
- Services provided
- Equipment
- Technology utilized

Observation

- Health care providers
- Team skills
- Communication skills
- Safety procedures
- Therapeutic/diagnostic procedures

Knowledge

- New information learned
- Medical terminology
- Skills learned

Evaluation

- Personal experience
- Educational value
- Professional value

Journal Entry

Write a journal entry summarizing your clinical experience.

____

____

____

____

____

____

Name ______________________ Date ____________ Period ____________

Pain Management Pre-Clinical Worksheet

Instructions: Answer the following questions.

1. Define the central nervous system.

____

____

2. Define the peripheral nervous system.

____

____

3. What are the main functions of the four major parts of the brain listed below?

A. Cerebrum:

____

____

B. Cerebellum:

____

____

C. Brain stem:

____

____

D. Diencephalon:

____

____

4. Identify the system and describe the function(s) of each of the cranial nerves.

A. Olfactory:

____

____

B. Optic:

____

____

C. Oculomotor:

____

____

(Continued)

D. Trochlear:

E. Trigeminal:

F. Abducens:

G. Facial:

H. Vestibulocochlear:

I. Glossopharyngeal:

J. Vagus:

K. Accessory:

L. Hypoglossal:

5. The thirty-one pairs of spinal nerves branch out from both the right and left sides of the spinal cord. Each pair is named for the vertebral level from which it originates and connects to the organ and tissues of the upper body and the limbs. Research the following nerves, then record their location and common issues that may occur if damaged.

   A. C4:

   B. T4:

(Continued)

Name ______________________________

C. T10:

____

____

D. L2:

____

____

E. L5/S1:

____

____

6. Describe the function of the autonomic nervous system:

____

____

7. Describe the function of the somatic nervous system:

____

____

8. Describe the function of the parasympathetic nervous system:

____

____

9. Define the following terms.

A. Acute pain:

____

____

B. Chronic pain:

____

____

C. Fibromyalgia:

____

____

D. Hyperpathia:

____

____

E. Peripheral neuropathy:

____

____

(Continued)

F. Traumatic brain injury (TBI):

G. Cerebral palsy:

H. Concussion:

I. Paraplegia:

J. Quadriplegia:

K. Hemiplegia:

L. Paresthesia:

M. Paralysis:

N. Tremor:

O. Unconscious:

10. Describe the following treatments.
    A. Analgesic:

    B. Anesthetic:

(Continued)

Name ______________________________

C. Cryotherapy:

____

____

D. Epidural:

____

____

E. Narcotic:

____

____

F. Nerve block:

____

____

G. NSAID:

____

____

H. Opioid:

____

____

I. Pharmacotherapy:

____

____

J. Patient controlled analgesia (PCA-pump):

____

____

K. Peripheral nerve block:

____

____

L. Trigger point injection:

____

____

M. Transcutaneous electrical nerve stimulation (TENS):

____

____

N. Stimulant:

____

____

Notes

Name ______________________ Date ____________ Period ____________

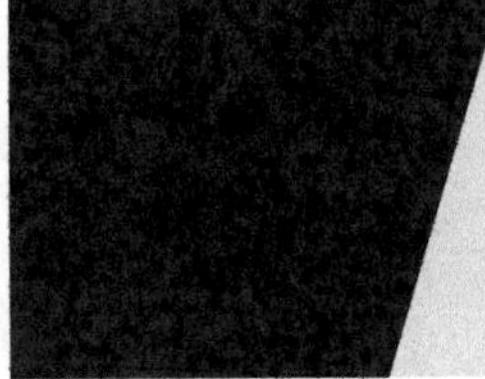

Pain Management Workplace Discovery Sheet

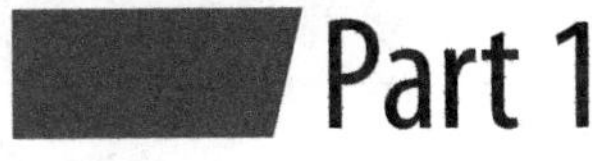

Part 1

During the Clinical Experience

Instructions: Answer the following questions.

1. What type of license/degree/credential is required for working in pain management?

____

____

2. Etiology of pain is generally divided into three main types: pain caused by tissue damage, pain caused by nerve damage and psychogenic pain. Which types of pain therapy does your department work with?

____

____

3. How is pain assessed and identified?

____

____

4. What is a pain scale?

____

____

5. Why is pain management important for the post-operative client?

____

____

6. What is the common method of pain management used for each of the following types of *acute* pain?

   A. Neck pain:

   ____

   ____

   B. Upper back pain:

   ____

   ____

   C. Lower back pain:

   ____

   ____

(Continued)

D. Shoulder pain:

E. Arm pain:

F. Hip pain:

G. Leg pain:

7. What is the common method of pain management used for each of the following types of *chronic* pain?

A. Neck pain:

B. Upper back pain:

C. Lower back pain:

D. Shoulder pain:

E. Arm pain:

F. Hip pain:

G. Leg pain:

8. How frequently are most clients with chronic pain seen by a pain management team?

(Continued)

Name ____________________

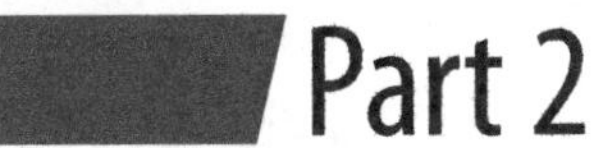

Part 2

After the Clinical Experience

Instructions: For each item below, identify whether you observed or assisted. Then, provide a brief summary.

Orientation

1. Equipment
   - ☐ Observed
   - ☐ Assisted

   Brief summary:

   ____

   ____

2. Standard precautions
   - ☐ Observed
   - ☐ Assisted

   Brief summary:

   ____

   ____

Pain Management Procedures

3. Facet block
   - ☐ Observed
   - ☐ Assisted

   Brief summary:

   ____

   ____

4. Nerve block to neck
   - ☐ Observed
   - ☐ Assisted

   Brief summary:

   ____

   ____

5. Facet with fluoroscopy
   - ☐ Observed
   - ☐ Assisted

   Brief summary:

   ____

   ____

(Continued)

6. Stelate ganglion block
   ☐ Observed
   ☐ Assisted
   Brief summary:

   ____

   ____

7. Trigger point injection
   ☐ Observed
   ☐ Assisted
   Brief summary:

   ____

   ____

8. Lumbar epidural injection
   ☐ Observed
   ☐ Assisted
   Brief summary:

   ____

   ____

9. Lumbar sympathetic block
   ☐ Observed
   ☐ Assisted
   Brief summary:

   ____

   ____

10. Follow up procedures
    ☐ Observed
    ☐ Assisted
    Brief summary:

    ____

    ____

Clinic Procedures

11. Assist client to room
    ☐ Observed
    ☐ Assisted
    Brief summary:

    ____

    ____

(Continued)

Name ____

12. Client history
    - ☐ Observed
    - ☐ Assisted

    Brief summary:

    ____

    ____

13. Client assessment
    - ☐ Observed
    - ☐ Assisted

    Brief summary:

    ____

    ____

14. Vital signs
    - ☐ Observed
    - ☐ Assisted

    Brief summary:

    ____

    ____

15. Room setup
    - ☐ Observed
    - ☐ Assisted

    Brief summary:

    ____

    ____

16. Instrument setup
    - ☐ Observed
    - ☐ Assisted

    Brief summary:

    ____

    ____

17. Client education
    - ☐ Observed
    - ☐ Assisted

    Brief summary:

    ____

    ____

(Continued)

18. Follow-up visits
    ☐ Observed
    ☐ Assisted
    Brief summary:

    ____

    ____

19. Client teaching
    ☐ Observed
    ☐ Assisted
    Brief summary:

    ____

    ____

Student Name: ______________________________

Technician Name: ____________________________

Student ______________________ Dates ____________ Site ____________ Preceptor ____________

Pain Management Post-Clinical Reflection

Rotation Report

Overview

Instructions: Answer the following questions using complete sentences.

1. What were your responsibilities or duties this week?

2. What new knowledge or skill did you learn or observe this week?

3. What was the best thing that happened at your clinical site this week?

4. What was the most challenging thing that happened at your clinical site this week?

5. What problems or difficulties did you encounter or observe at your clinical site? How were they dealt with?

6. Was this week good, fair, or bad? Explain.

Observations

Instructions: List the observations you made for each of the following categories.

1. Technology observed:

2. Diagnostic procedures observed:

(Continued)

3. Therapeutic procedures observed:

____

____

4. Diseases or disorders observed:

____

____

5. Medical terminology or abbreviations encountered:

____

____

6. Other observations:

____

____

Supervisor Signature: ______________________

Date: ______________________

Rotation Journal

Instructions: Write a journal entry detailing your learning experience at the clinical rotation. Use the following topics to help write a complete journal entry.

Assessment of the Environment

- Personnel
- Services provided
- Equipment
- Technology utilized

Observation

- Health care providers
- Team skills
- Communication skills
- Safety procedures
- Therapeutic/diagnostic procedures

Knowledge

- New information learned
- Medical terminology
- Skills learned

Evaluation

- Personal experience
- Educational value
- Professional value

Journal Entry

Write a journal entry summarizing your clinical experience.

____

____

____

____

____

____

Name ______________________ Date ____________ Period ____________

Pediatrics Pre-Clinical Worksheet

Instructions: Answer the following questions.

1. Define the following terms.

   A. Infancy:

   B. Early childhood:

   C. Middle childhood:

   D. Late childhood:

   E. Adolescence:

   F. Physical growth:

   G. Mental growth:

   H. Emotional growth:

   I. Social growth:

   J. Client advocate:

(Continued)

2. Describe the major physical development found in each of the following stages.

A. Infancy:

B. Early childhood:

C. Middle childhood:

D. Late childhood:

E. Adolescence:

3. Describe what normal social development looks like in the following stages.

A. Early childhood:

B. Middle childhood:

C. Late childhood:

D. Adolescence:

4. What type of growth does play therapy target?

5. What are the three basic functions of play therapy?

(Continued)

Name ____________________

6. What is a child life specialist's goal in a hospital/healthcare setting?

7. Describe the following disorders.
   A. Autism:

   B. ADHD:

   C. Cerebral palsy:

   D. Celiacs:

   E. Cystic fibrosis:

   F. Sickle cell anemia:

   G. Juvenile diabetes:

   H. Epiglottitis:

   I. Appendicitis:

   J. Idiopathic thrombocytopenia:

   K. Acute lymphocytic leukemia:

(Continued)

L. Asthma:

M. Dehydration:

8. What is Early Childhood Intervention (ECI)?

9. What age group does ECI include?

10. What is the purpose of ECI?

11. Who is eligible for ECI?

12. What is the coverage area for Betty Hardwick ECI?

13. What is the Mission Statement for Betty Hardwick Center?

14. What are their values?

15. What is MHFA?

16. Who is the MHFA coordinator for Betty Hardwick?

(Continued)

Name ______________________________

17. Define the following terms.
    A. Disability:

    B. Developmental delay:

    C. Cognitive delay:

    D. Crisis respite care:

    E. Crisis intervention:

18. Describe the first aid treatment for a closed fracture of the arm or leg.

19. What is the leading cause (microorganism) of strep throat?

20. What type of health screenings might occur at school?

21. Describe the common symptoms of the following disorders.
    A. Strep throat:

    B. Mild concussion:

    C. Ear infection:

(Continued)

D. COVID-19:

E. RSV:

F. Hand-foot-mouth-disease:

G. Head lice:

H. Mononucleosis:

I. Sinusitis:

J. Whooping cough:

K. Norovirus:

L. Chickenpox:

M. Meningitis:

Name ______________________ Date ____________ Period ____________

Pediatrics Workplace Discovery Sheet

Part 1

During the Clinical Experience

Instructions: Answer the following questions.

1. How many different staff members work in the clinic?

2. What are the educational requirements for the different staff members?

3. What additional courses do you wish you had taken in high school or college to be more prepared for this field of work?

4. What do you like most about this career? Dislike?

5. How many clients do you see on a daily basis?

6. What type of toys are used in play therapy for a toddler/preschooler? For school-age child? (List at least three for each.)

7. What types of therapies are used with teens?

(Continued)

8. What extra safety measures are followed in pediatrics?

9. What are visitation restrictions on a pediatric unit?

10. What are the signs and symptoms of a child in respiratory distress?

11. What are the signs and symptoms of a child with dehydration?

12. What is the recommended pediatric vaccination schedule?

13. What extra safety measures are followed in the classroom for a student with disabilities?

14. What is the procedure for tube feeding at the school?

15. What are the common signs of hypoglycemia and what is the protocol for a blood sugar that is abnormally low?

16. What are the common signs of hyperglycemia and what is the protocol for a blood sugar that is abnormally high?

17. What is the protocol if a student is found to have pediculosis capitis?

18. Why do you think inclusion is important for a child with disabilities?

(Continued)

Name ____________________

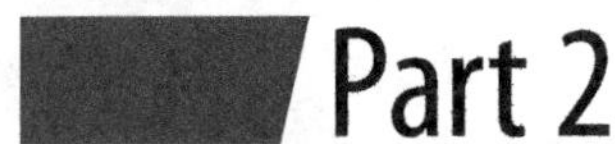

Part 2

After the Clinical Experience

Instructions: For each item below, identify whether you observed or assisted. Then, provide a brief summary.

Play Therapy Preparation to Relieve Client Anxiety Before a Procedure

1. Toddler
   - ☐ Observed
   - ☐ Assisted

   Brief summary:

   ____

   ____

2. School-age child
   - ☐ Observed
   - ☐ Assisted

   Brief summary:

   ____

   ____

3. Adolescent
   - ☐ Observed
   - ☐ Assisted

   Brief summary:

   ____

   ____

Play Therapy Activities

4. For language development
   - ☐ Observed
   - ☐ Assisted

   Brief summary:

   ____

   ____

5. For eye-hand coordination
   - ☐ Observed
   - ☐ Assisted

   Brief summary:

   ____

   ____

(Continued)

6. For mental stimulation
   ☐ Observed
   ☐ Assisted
   Brief summary:

   ____

   ____

7. Developmental stages
   ☐ Observed
   ☐ Assisted
   Brief summary:

   ____

   ____

8. Behavior reinforcement
   ☐ Observed
   ☐ Assisted
   Brief summary:

   ____

   ____

9. Managing behavioral issues
   ☐ Observed
   ☐ Assisted
   Brief summary:

   ____

   ____

Human Relations

10. Staff interaction
    ☐ Observed
    ☐ Assisted
    Brief summary:

    ____

    ____

11. Child-parent interaction
    ☐ Observed
    ☐ Assisted
    Brief summary:

    ____

    ____

(Continued)

Name ____

Pediatrics

12. Assessment/vital signs
    - ☐ Observed
    - ☐ Assisted

    Brief summary:

    ____

    ____

13. Height and weight measurement
    - ☐ Observed
    - ☐ Assisted

    Brief summary:

    ____

    ____

14. Intake and output
    - ☐ Observed
    - ☐ Assisted

    Brief summary:

    ____

    ____

15. Bathing and AM care
    - ☐ Observed
    - ☐ Assisted

    Brief summary:

    ____

    ____

16. Universal precautions
    - ☐ Observed
    - ☐ Assisted

    Brief summary:

    ____

    ____

17. Medication administration
    - ☐ Observed
    - ☐ Assisted

    Brief summary:

    ____

    ____

(Continued)

Nutrition

18. Meals/formulas
    - ☐ Observed
    - ☐ Assisted

    Brief summary:

    ____

    ____

19. Nutritional requirements
    - ☐ Observed
    - ☐ Assisted

    Brief summary:

    ____

    ____

20. Special diets
    - ☐ Observed
    - ☐ Assisted

    Brief summary:

    ____

    ____

Adjustment to the Clinical/School Setting

21. Fear reduction
    - ☐ Observed
    - ☐ Assisted

    Brief summary:

    ____

    ____

22. Promotion of trust
    - ☐ Observed
    - ☐ Assisted

    Brief summary:

    ____

    ____

23. Parental support
    - ☐ Observed
    - ☐ Assisted

    Brief summary:

    ____

    ____

(Continued)

Name ______________________________

24. Emergency care
    - ☐ Observed
    - ☐ Assisted

    Brief summary:

    ____

    ____

Manifestation/Management of Health Conditions

25. Orthopedic injuries
    - ☐ Observed
    - ☐ Assisted

    Brief summary:

    ____

    ____

26. Respiratory diseases/disorders
    - ☐ Observed
    - ☐ Assisted

    Brief summary:

    ____

    ____

27. Congenital anomalies
    - ☐ Observed
    - ☐ Assisted

    Brief summary:

    ____

    ____

28. Medical conditions
    - ☐ Observed
    - ☐ Assisted

    Brief summary:

    ____

    ____

Client Services

29. Client screening and assessment
    - ☐ Observed
    - ☐ Assisted

    Brief summary:

    ____

    ____

(Continued)

30. Client admission and discharge procedures

☐ Observed

☐ Assisted

Brief summary:

____

____

31. Medical services

☐ Observed

☐ Assisted

Brief summary:

____

____

Assistive Technology

32. Services

☐ Observed

☐ Assisted

Brief summary:

____

____

33. Devices

☐ Observed

☐ Assisted

Brief summary:

____

____

Counseling

34. Family counseling

☐ Observed

☐ Assisted

Brief summary:

____

____

35. Individual counseling

☐ Observed

☐ Assisted

Brief summary:

____

____

(Continued)

Name ____

36. Group counseling
    ☐ Observed
    ☐ Assisted
    Brief summary:

    ____

    ____

Therapy

37. Physical therapy
    ☐ Observed
    ☐ Assisted
    Brief summary:

    ____

    ____

38. Occupational therapy
    ☐ Observed
    ☐ Assisted
    Brief summary:

    ____

    ____

39. Speech-language therapy
    ☐ Observed
    ☐ Assisted
    Brief summary:

    ____

    ____

40. Behavioral therapy
    ☐ Observed
    ☐ Assisted
    Brief summary:

    ____

    ____

Classroom

41. Inclusion
    ☐ Observed
    ☐ Assisted
    Brief summary:

    ____

    ____

(Continued)

42. Modifications
    ☐ Observed
    ☐ Assisted
    Brief summary:

    ____

    ____

43. Private duty nurse
    ☐ Observed
    ☐ Assisted
    Brief summary:

    ____

    ____

44. Teaching strategies
    ☐ Observed
    ☐ Assisted
    Brief summary:

    ____

    ____

Student Name: ______________________________

Technician Name: ____________ ______________

Student ________________ Dates ________ Site ________ Preceptor ________

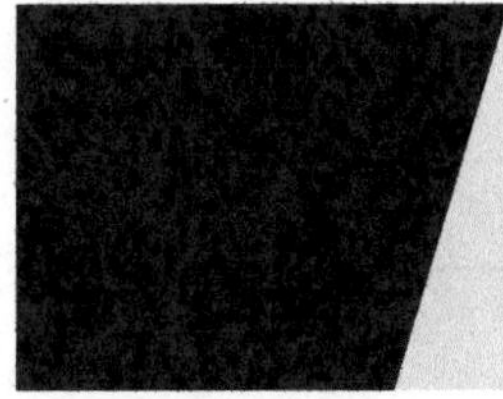

Pediatrics Post-Clinical Reflection

Rotation Report

Overview

Instructions: Answer the following questions using complete sentences.

1. What were your responsibilities or duties this week?

____

____

2. What new knowledge or skill did you learn or observe this week?

____

____

3. What was the best thing that happened at your clinical site this week?

____

____

4. What was the most challenging thing that happened at your clinical site this week?

____

____

5. What problems or difficulties did you encounter or observe at your clinical site? How were they dealt with?

____

____

6. Was this week good, fair, or bad? Explain.

____

____

Observations

Instructions: List the observations you made for each of the following categories.

1. Technology observed:

____

____

2. Diagnostic procedures observed:

____

____

(Continued)

3. Therapeutic procedures observed:

____

____

4. Diseases or disorders observed:

____

____

5. Medical terminology or abbreviations encountered:

____

____

6. Other observations:

____

____

Supervisor Signature: ______________________________

Date: ______________________________

Rotation Journal

Instructions: Write a journal entry detailing your learning experience at the clinical rotation. Use the following topics to help write a complete journal entry.

Assessment of the Environment

- Personnel
- Services provided
- Equipment
- Technology utilized

Observation

- Health care providers
- Team skills
- Communication skills
- Safety procedures
- Therapeutic/diagnostic procedures

Knowledge

- New information learned
- Medical terminology
- Skills learned

Evaluation

- Personal experience
- Educational value
- Professional value

Journal Entry

Write a journal entry summarizing your clinical experience.

____

____

____

____

____

____

Name ______________________ Date ____________ Period __________

Pharmacy Pre-Clinical Worksheet

Instructions: Answer the following questions.

1. Define the word *pharmacology*.

____

____

2. Describe the following terms associated with the drug cycle.

   A. Absorption:

   ____

   ____

   B. Distribution:

   ____

   ____

   C. Metabolism:

   ____

   ____

   D. Excretion:

   ____

   ____

3. What is a medication that causes stimulation of a receptors called?

____

4. What is a medication that binds to a receptor and blocks other medication called?

____

5. Define the following terms as they pertain to drugs.

   A. Dose:

   ____

   ____

   B. Action:

   ____

   ____

   C. Side effects:

   ____

   ____

(Continued)

D. Contraindication:

E. Generic name:

F. Trade name:

G. OTC:

6. Describe the following routes of drug administration.
   A. Enteral medications:

   B. Parenteral medications:

   C. Rectal:

   D. Oral:

   E. Buccal:

   F. Intravenous:

   G. Intraosseous:

   H. Subcutaneous:

(Continued)

Name ____________________

I. Intramuscular:

____

____

J. Inhalation:

____

____

K. Sublingual:

____

____

L. Transdermal:

____

____

M. Intranasal:

____

____

7. Describe the following medication forms.

A. Tablet:

____

____

B. Capsule:

____

____

C. Solution:

____

____

D. Suspension:

____

____

E. Meter dose inhaler:

____

____

F. Lotion:

____

____

G. Cream:

____

____

(Continued)

H. Ointment:

I. Patch:

J. Gels:

K. Pellet:

8. What are the six rights of medication administration?

9. Research acetaminophen and record the following information about it.
   A. Trade/brand name:

   B. Action:

   C. Indication:

   D. Contraindications:

   E. Routes:

   F. Side effects:

   G. Interactions:

(Continued)

Name ____

H. Dose for adults:

____

____

I. Doses for children under the age of twelve:

____

____

J. Doses for infants:

____

____

10. What does the term *drug classification* mean?

____

____

11. What does the term *hypersensitivity* mean?

____

____

12. Translate the following doctor's orders:

A. Lipitor 10 mg
Sig: po qd @ hs
Disp: 90 tablets

____

____

B. Cyclobenzaprine 10 mg
Sig: po tid x 10 days
Disp: 30 tablets

____

____

Notes

Name ______________________ Date ____________ Period ____________

Pharmacy Workplace Discovery Sheet

Part 1

During the Clinical Experience

Instructions: Answer the following questions.

1. Describe the educational and licensing difference between a pharmacist and pharmacy technician.

2. List the seven parts of a prescription.

3. Describe the difference between a brand name and a generic drug.

4. What are the five rights of medication dispensing?

5. What four pieces of information must a pharmacist have to dispense a refill?

6. What is the procedure for handling the transfer of a prescription from one pharmacy to another?

7. What do the *X* marks on bottles/containers on the shelves mean?

8. What happens to medications that are going to expire or are already expired?

(Continued)

9. What client information is needed to fill a prescription?

10. Translate the following abbreviations used in the pharmacy:

   A. Rx:

   B. PR:

   C. PO:

   D. IV:

   E. IO:

   F. SC:

   G. IM:

   H. SL:

   I. Qd:

   J. BID:

   K. TID:

   L. QID:

   M. Q4h:

   N. Ac:

   O. Pc:

   P. OS:

(Continued)

Name ______________________________

Q. OD:

____

R. OU:

____

S. PRN:

____

T. STAT:

____

U. OTC:

____

Part 2

After the Clinical Experience

Instructions: For each item below, identify whether you observed or assisted. Then, provide a brief summary.

Procedures

1. Charging/billing/credit
   - ☐ Observed
   - ☐ Assisted

   Brief summary:

   ____

   ____

2. Use of pharmacy profile
   - ☐ Observed
   - ☐ Assisted

   Brief summary:

   ____

   ____

3. Inventory
   - ☐ Observed
   - ☐ Assisted

   Brief summary:

   ____

   ____

(Continued)

4. Reconciliation
   - ☐ Observed
   - ☐ Assisted

   Brief summary:

   ____

   ____

5. Narcotic tracking methods
   - ☐ Observed
   - ☐ Assisted

   Brief summary:

   ____

   ____

Filling Medication Orders

6. Accuracy quality checks
   - ☐ Observed
   - ☐ Assisted

   Brief summary:

   ____

   ____

7. Dosage calculation
   - ☐ Observed
   - ☐ Assisted

   Brief summary:

   ____

   ____

8. Medication order
   - ☐ Observed
   - ☐ Assisted

   Brief summary:

   ____

   ____

9. Medication distribution
   - ☐ Observed
   - ☐ Assisted

   Brief summary:

   ____

   ____

(Continued)

Name ______________________________

Services

10. Emergency floor stock
    - ☐ Observed
    - ☐ Assisted

    Brief summary:

    ____

    ____

11. Crash cart medications
    - ☐ Observed
    - ☐ Assisted

    Brief summary:

    ____

    ____

Other

12. IV medication preparation techniques
    - ☐ Observed
    - ☐ Assisted

    Brief summary:

    ____

    ____

13. Technology
    - ☐ Observed
    - ☐ Assisted

    Brief summary:

    ____

    ____

14. Handling of emergencies
    - ☐ Observed
    - ☐ Assisted

    Brief summary:

    ____

    ____

(Continued)

15. Client teaching/education
    ☐ Observed
    ☐ Assisted
    Brief summary:

    ____

    ____

Student Name: ________________________________

Technician Name: ______________________________

Student ______________________ Dates ____________ Site ____________ Preceptor ____________

Pharmacy Post-Clinical Reflection

Rotation Report

Overview

Instructions: Answer the following questions using complete sentences.

1. What were your responsibilities or duties this week?

2. What new knowledge or skill did you learn or observe this week?

3. What was the best thing that happened at your clinical site this week?

4. What was the most challenging thing that happened at your clinical site this week?

5. What problems or difficulties did you encounter or observe at your clinical site? How were they dealt with?

6. Was this week good, fair, or bad? Explain.

Observations

Instructions: List the observations you made for each of the following categories.

1. Technology observed:

2. Diagnostic procedures observed:

(Continued)

3. Therapeutic procedures observed:

____

____

4. Diseases or disorders observed:

____

____

5. Medical terminology or abbreviations encountered:

____

____

6. Other observations:

____

____

Supervisor Signature: ______________________________

Date: ______________________________

Rotation Journal

Instructions: Write a journal entry detailing your learning experience at the clinical rotation. Use the following topics to help write a complete journal entry.

Assessment of the Environment

- Personnel
- Services provided
- Equipment
- Technology utilized

Observation

- Health care providers
- Team skills
- Communication skills
- Safety procedures
- Therapeutic/diagnostic procedures

Knowledge

- New information learned
- Medical terminology
- Skills learned

Evaluation

- Personal experience
- Educational value
- Professional value

Journal Entry

Write a journal entry summarizing your clinical experience.

____

____

____

____

____

____

Name ______________________ Date ____________ Period ____________

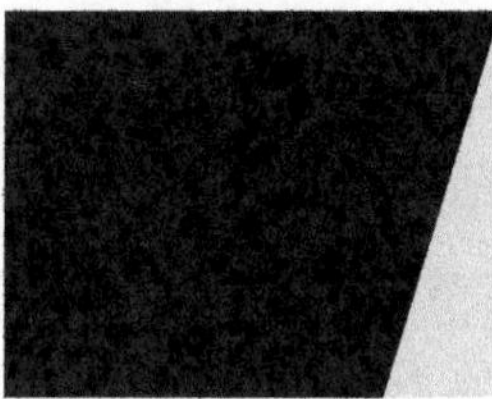

Physician's Office Pre-Clinical Worksheet

Instructions: Answer the following questions.

1. Define the following terms.

   A. Acute:

   ____

   ____

   B. Chronic:

   ____

   ____

   C. Congenital:

   ____

   ____

   D. Genetic:

   ____

   ____

   E. Hypersensitivity:

   ____

   ____

   F. Idiopathic:

   ____

   ____

   G. Infectious:

   ____

   ____

   H. Malaise:

   ____

   ____

   I. Prophylaxis:

   ____

   ____

   J. Syndrome:

   ____

   ____

(Continued)

K. Neglect:

L. Epiphyseal plate:

M. Vaccination:

2. Define the following conditions.

A. H/A:

B. Influenza:

C. Concussion:

D. Laceration:

E. HFMD:

F. Pediculosis capitis:

G. Pertussis:

H. Impetigo:

I. Norovirus:

(Continued)

Name ______________________________

J. Rheumatic arthritis:

____

____

K. Conjunctivitis:

____

____

L. Rhinovirus:

____

____

3. Describe the differences between these types of fractures below.
   A. Comminuted:

____

____

   B. Compression:

____

____

   C. Greenstick:

____

____

   D. Longitudinal:

____

____

   E. Oblique:

____

____

   F. Spiral:

____

____

   G. Transverse:

____

____

   H. Open:

____

____

   I. Closed:

____

____

(Continued)

4. Describe the common symptoms of the following disorders.
   A. Strep throat:

   ______

   ______

   B. Mild concussion:

   ______

   ______

   C. Ear infection:

   ______

   ______

   D. COVID-19:

   ______

   ______

   E. RSV:

   ______

   ______

   F. Hand-foot-mouth-disease:

   ______

   ______

   G. Head lice:

   ______

   ______

   H. Mononucleosis:

   ______

   ______

   I. Sinusitis:

   ______

   ______

   J. Whooping cough:

   ______

   ______

   K. Norovirus:

   ______

   ______

(Continued)

Name ______________________________

L. Chickenpox:

____

____

M. Meningitis:

____

____

Notes

Name ______________________ Date ____________ Period ____________

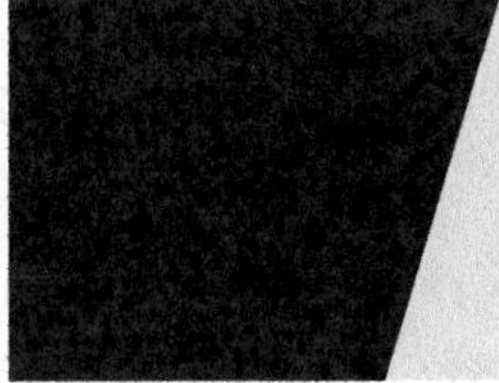

Physician's Office Workplace Discovery Sheet

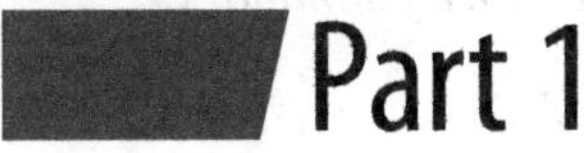

Part 1

During the Clinical Experience

Instructions: Answer the following questions.

1. What are the types of careers and educational requirements needed for the professionals who work in a physician's office?

2. What are the requirements to maintain licensure as a physician?

3. Are there any challenges related to the practice in setting?

4. What is the average number of clients seen daily in the clinic?

5. What is the most common condition seen in the clinic?

6. What is the most challenging condition to treat?

7. What does a normal day look like in this profession?

8. What type of preventative teaching is given to clients?

(Continued)

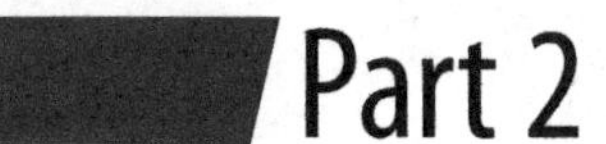

Part 2

After the Clinical Experience

Instructions: For each item below, identify whether you observed or assisted. Then, provide a brief summary.

Information Handling and Processing

1. Assembling records

   ☐ Observed

   ☐ Assisted

   Brief summary:

   ____

   ____

2. Legal acceptances

   ☐ Observed

   ☐ Assisted

   Brief summary:

   ____

   ____

3. Client's right to information

   ☐ Observed

   ☐ Assisted

   Brief summary:

   ____

   ____

4. Release of information

   ☐ Observed

   ☐ Assisted

   Brief summary:

   ____

   ____

5. Confidentiality

   ☐ Observed

   ☐ Assisted

   Brief summary:

   ____

   ____

(Continued)

Name ________________________________

Checking a Client In

6. Vision exam
   - ☐ Observed
   - ☐ Assisted

   Brief summary:

   ____

   ____

7. Height and weight
   - ☐ Observed
   - ☐ Assisted

   Brief summary:

   ____

   ____

8. Taking client to exam room
   - ☐ Observed
   - ☐ Assisted

   Brief summary:

   ____

   ____

9. Obtaining vital signs
   - ☐ Observed
   - ☐ Assisted

   Brief summary:

   ____

   ____

10. Assisting with exam
    - ☐ Observed
    - ☐ Assisted

    Brief summary:

    ____

    ____

Numbering and Filing Records

11. Organizational patterns
    - ☐ Observed
    - ☐ Assisted

    Brief summary:

    ____

    ____

(Continued)

12. Coding and indexing systems

☐ Observed

☐ Assisted

Brief summary:

____

____

13. Other records/documents

☐ Observed

☐ Assisted

Brief summary:

____

____

Manifestation/Management of Health Conditions

14. Orthopedic injuries

☐ Observed

☐ Assisted

Brief summary:

____

____

15. Respiratory diseases/disorders

☐ Observed

☐ Assisted

Brief summary:

____

____

16. Congenital anomalies

☐ Observed

☐ Assisted

Brief summary:

____

____

17. Medical conditions

☐ Observed

☐ Assisted

Brief summary:

____

____

Student Name: ______________________________

Technician Name: ____________________________

Student ______________________ Dates ____________ Site ____________ Preceptor ____________

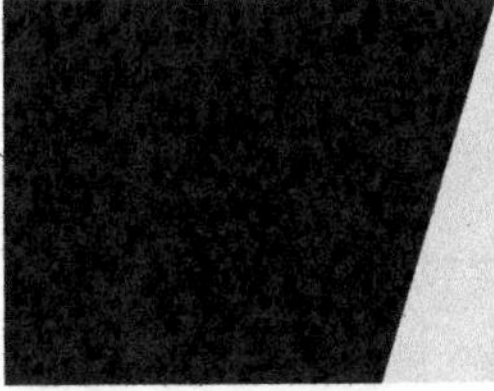

Physician's Office Post-Clinical Reflection

Rotation Report

Overview

Instructions: Answer the following questions using complete sentences.

1. What were your responsibilities or duties this week?

____

____

2. What new knowledge or skill did you learn or observe this week?

____

____

3. What was the best thing that happened at your clinical site this week?

____

____

4. What was the most challenging thing that happened at your clinical site this week?

____

____

5. What problems or difficulties did you encounter or observe at your clinical site? How were they dealt with?

____

____

6. Was this week good, fair, or bad? Explain.

____

____

Observations

Instructions: List the observations you made for each of the following categories.

1. Technology observed:

____

____

2. Diagnostic procedures observed:

____

____

(Continued)

3. Therapeutic procedures observed:

____

____

4. Diseases or disorders observed:

____

____

5. Medical terminology or abbreviations encountered:

____

____

6. Other observations:

____

____

Supervisor Signature: ______________________________

Date: ______________________________

Rotation Journal

Instructions: Write a journal entry detailing your learning experience at the clinical rotation. Use the following topics to help write a complete journal entry.

Assessment of the Environment

- Personnel
- Services provided
- Equipment
- Technology utilized

Observation

- Health care providers
- Team skills
- Communication skills
- Safety procedures
- Therapeutic/diagnostic procedures

Knowledge

- New information learned
- Medical terminology
- Skills learned

Evaluation

- Personal experience
- Educational value
- Professional value

Journal Entry

Write a journal entry summarizing your clinical experience.

____

____

____

____

____

____

Name ______________________ Date __________ Period __________

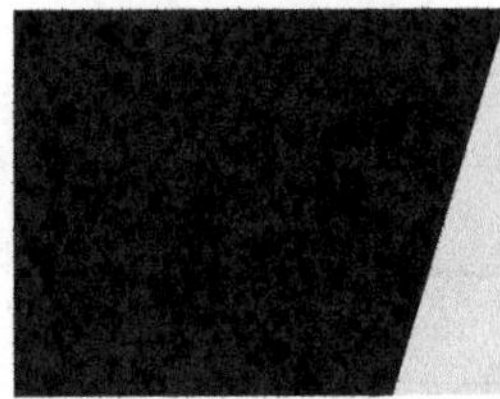

Psychology Pre-Clinical Worksheet

Instructions: Answer the following questions.

1. What services does a psychology center offer?

2. What is psychotherapy? What are the alternative names of this therapy?

3. How can culture and social factors affect human behavior?

4. How can the brain and biology impact behavior?

5. Describe risk factors of behavior common in adolescence.

6. What is meant by the phrase "nature vs nurture"?

7. How do you think childhood events can influence later mental health?

(Continued)

8. What do you think are some of the challenges you would encounter working in a mental health career path?

9. Define the following terms related to psychology.
   A. Anxiety:

   B. Mindfulness:

   C. Coping mechanism:

   D. Defense mechanism:

   E. Delusion:

   F. Self-efficacy:

   G. Hierarchy of needs:

Name ______________________ Date ______________ Period ____________

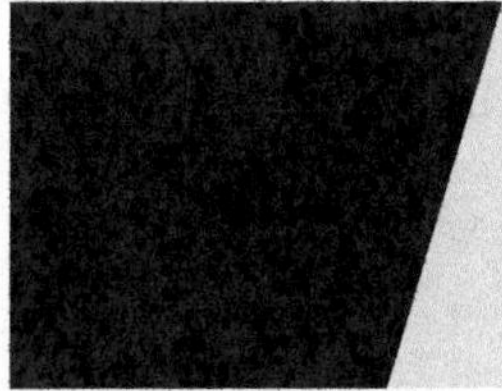

Psychology Workplace Discovery Sheet

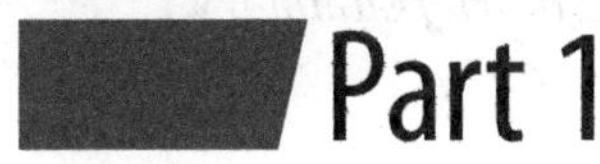

Part 1

During the Clinical Experience

Instructions: Answer the following questions.

1. What are the types of careers and educational requirements needed for professionals who work in a psychology office?

2. What are the requirements to maintain licensure in psychology?

3. Are there any challenges related to the practice in psychology?

4. What is the average number of clients seen daily in the psychology clinic?

5. What is the most common condition seen in the clinic?

6. What is the most challenging condition to treat?

7. What does a normal day look like in this profession?

8. What type of preventative teaching does psychology treatment provide?

(Continued)

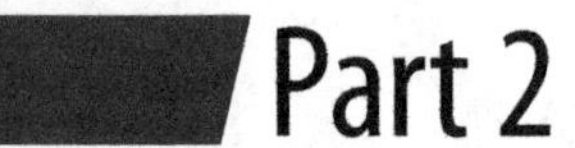 Part 2

After the Clinical Experience

Instructions: For each item below, identify whether you observed or assisted. Then, provide a brief summary.

Client Services

1. Client screening
   ☐ Observed
   ☐ Assisted
   Brief summary:
   ____
   ____

2. Client assessment
   ☐ Observed
   ☐ Assisted
   Brief summary:
   ____
   ____

3. Client admission
   ☐ Observed
   ☐ Assisted
   Brief summary:
   ____
   ____

4. Emergency procedures
   ☐ Observed
   ☐ Assisted
   Brief summary:
   ____
   ____

5. Discharge procedures
   ☐ Observed
   ☐ Assisted
   Brief summary:
   ____
   ____

(Continued)

Name ____

6. Psychological services
   - ☐ Observed
   - ☐ Assisted

   Brief summary:

   ____

   ____

7. Social work services
   - ☐ Observed
   - ☐ Assisted

   Brief summary:

   ____

   ____

Counseling

8. Family counseling
   - ☐ Observed
   - ☐ Assisted

   Brief summary:

   ____

   ____

9. Individual counseling
   - ☐ Observed
   - ☐ Assisted

   Brief summary:

   ____

   ____

10. Group counseling
    - ☐ Observed
    - ☐ Assisted

    Brief summary:

    ____

    ____

(Continued)

Therapy Offered

11. Therapy type #1

    Type:

    ____

    ☐ Observed

    ☐ Assisted

    Brief summary:

    ____

    ____

12. Therapy type #2

    Type:

    ____

    ☐ Observed

    ☐ Assisted

    Brief summary:

    ____

    ____

13. Therapy type #3

    Type:

    ____

    ☐ Observed

    ☐ Assisted

    Brief summary:

    ____

    ____

Prevention Services

14. Prevention services type #1

    Type:

    ____

    ☐ Observed

    ☐ Assisted

    Brief summary:

    ____

    ____

(Continued)

Name ____

15. Prevention services type #2

Type:

____

☐ Observed

☐ Assisted

Brief summary:

____

____

16. Prevention services type #3

Type:

____

☐ Observed

☐ Assisted

Brief summary:

____

____

Resources

17. Resource type #1

Type:

____

☐ Observed

☐ Assisted

Brief summary:

____

____

18. Resource type #2

Type:

____

☐ Observed

☐ Assisted

Brief summary:

____

____

(Continued)

19. Resource type #3

Type:

____

☐ Observed

☐ Assisted

Brief summary:

____

____

Other

20. Confidentiality

☐ Observed

☐ Assisted

Brief summary:

____

____

Student Name: ________________________________

Technician Name: ______________________________

Student ______________________ Dates ____________ Site ____________ Preceptor ____________

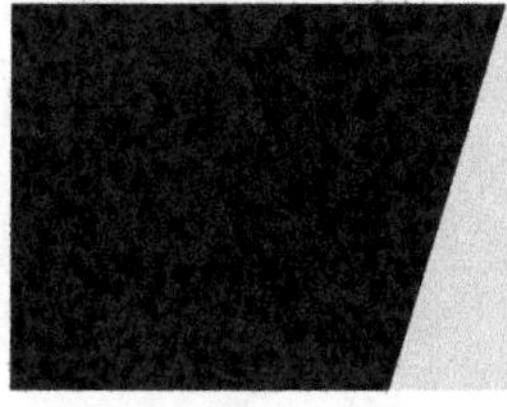

Psychology Post-Clinical Reflection

Rotation Report

Overview

Instructions: Answer the following questions using complete sentences.

1. What were your responsibilities or duties this week?

2. What new knowledge or skill did you learn or observe this week?

3. What was the best thing that happened at your clinical site this week?

4. What was the most challenging thing that happened at your clinical site this week?

5. What problems or difficulties did you encounter or observe at your clinical site? How were they dealt with?

6. Was this week good, fair, or bad? Explain.

Observations

Instructions: List the observations you made for each of the following categories.

1. Technology observed:

2. Diagnostic procedures observed:

(Continued)

3. Therapeutic procedures observed:

____

____

4. Diseases or disorders observed:

____

____

5. Medical terminology or abbreviations encountered:

____

____

6. Other observations:

____

____

Supervisor Signature: ______________________________

Date: ______________________________

Rotation Journal

Instructions: Write a journal entry detailing your learning experience at the clinical rotation. Use the following topics to help write a complete journal entry.

Assessment of the Environment

- Personnel
- Services provided
- Equipment
- Technology utilized

Observation

- Health care providers
- Team skills
- Communication skills
- Safety procedures
- Therapeutic/diagnostic procedures

Knowledge

- New information learned
- Medical terminology
- Skills learned

Evaluation

- Personal experience
- Educational value
- Professional value

Journal Entry

Write a journal entry summarizing your clinical experience.

____

____

____

____

____

____

Name ______________________ Date ____________ Period ____________

Radiology Services Pre-Clinical Worksheet

Instructions: Answer the following questions.

1. Differentiate between an MRI and a CAT/CT scan.

2. How does a sonogram or ultrasound procedure work?

3. How is ultrasound utilized during an amniocentesis?

4. What is ultrasound looking for on a gallbladder scan?

5. What is vascular ultrasound?

6. How is a venogram different from a vascular ultrasound?

7. What is radiation therapy used for?

8. What are the risks involved in using radiation therapy?

9. Interpret the following abbreviations:
   A. CRIF:

   B. DJD:

(Continued)

C. L, Lt:

D. LBP:

E. L5-S1:

F. ORIF:

G. R, Rt:

H. CXR:

I. CT:

J. MRI:

10. Starting at the mouth/oral cavity, list, in order, the parts of the alimentary canal that food travels.

11. Define the following signs and symptoms:
    A. Anorexia:

    B. Ascites:

    C. Aspiration:

    D. Borborygmus:

    E. Constipation:

(Continued)

Name ______________________________

F. Dehydration:

____

____

G. Diarrhea:

____

____

H. Dyspepsia:

____

____

I. Dysphagia:

____

____

J. Emesis:

____

____

K. Eructation:

____

____

L. Flatus:

____

____

M. Halitosis:

____

____

N. Hematemesis:

____

____

O. Hematochezia:

____

____

P. Jaundice:

____

____

Q. Nausea:

____

____

(Continued)

R. Polyp:

S. Reflux:

T. Regurgitation:

U. Ulcer:

12. Research the following disorders/diseases. Briefly describe the disorder and list the common signs and symptoms as well as treatments.
    A. Celiac disease:

    B. Cholecystitis:

    C. Cholelithiasis:

    D. Cirrhosis:

    E. Colon cancer:

    F. Crohn's disease:

    G. Diverticulosis:

(Continued)

Name ____

H. Esophageal varices:

I. GERD:

J. Hemorrhoids:

K. Hepatitis:

L. Hiatal hernia:

M. Inguinal hernia:

N. Ileus:

O. Intestinal adhesions:

P. Intussusception:

Q. Strangulating obstruction:

R. Volvulus:

S. Irritable bowel syndrome (IBS):

(Continued)

T. Peptic ulcer:

U. Ulcerative colitis:

13. Identify four common causes of a GI bleed

14. Identify three common acid blockers.

15. How does a laxative work?

16. Interpret the following abbreviations:
    A. ac, a.c.:

    B. BM:

    C. BS:

    D. EGD:

    E. NPO:

    F. N/V:

    G. SOB:

Name ______________________ Date ____________ Period ____________

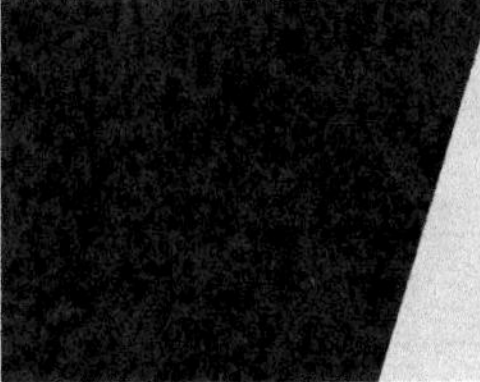

Radiology Services Workplace Discovery Sheet

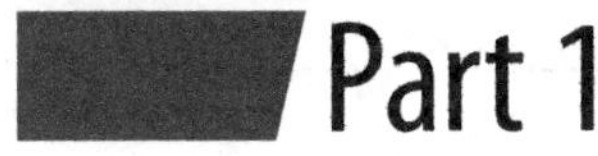

Part 1

During the Clinical Experience

Instructions: Answer the following questions.

1. What type of surgical procedures does the medical imaging department assist in?

2. What is the procedure for bringing a client down to X-ray who has been in isolation? In reverse isolation?

3. What is the most common X-ray performed?

4. Is there a radiologist available 24/7 to read X-rays?

5. With most X-ray information being transferred to the computer, are radiologists able to read a scan and make a report from home?

6. What types of X-rays require contrast media?

7. How are clients given radioactive substances for visualization?

8. What safety requirements are in place to protect health care providers from excessive radiation?

(Continued)

9. Describe the educational requirements and job duties for each of the following careers.
   A. Radiology technologist:

   B. Nuclear medical technologist:

   C. Radiation therapy technologist:

   D. Diagnostic medical sonographer:

10. Are clients who require radiation therapy in-client, out-client, or both?

11. For clients receiving radiation therapy, is there a standard number of treatments they normally must receive for certain conditions?

12. What are the typical pre-procedure instructions given to clients?

13. What type of anesthesia is used for esophagoscopies, colonoscopies, EGDs, proctoscopies, sigmoidoscopies, and fluoroscopies?

14. What organ biopsy procedures are typically done in this department and how common are they?

15. Describe the difference between a flexible and rigid endoscope.

16. Are there any types of treatment procedures that can be done during an endoscope?

(Continued)

Name ____

17. What are the common side effects of local, sedation, and general anesthesia?

____

____

18. What are common post-endoscopy instructions given to out-clients before dismissal?

____

____

Part 2

After the Clinical Experience

Instructions: For each item below, identify whether you observed or assisted. Then, provide a brief summary.

Orientation

1. Medical imaging
   - ☐ Observed
   - ☐ Assisted

   Brief summary:

   ____

   ____

2. Endoscopy lab
   - ☐ Observed
   - ☐ Assisted

   Brief summary:

   ____

   ____

Ultrasound Procedures

3. Gallbladder scan
   - ☐ Observed
   - ☐ Assisted

   Brief summary:

   ____

   ____

(Continued)

4. Renal scan
   ☐ Observed
   ☐ Assisted
   Brief summary:

   ____

   ____

5. Liver scan
   ☐ Observed
   ☐ Assisted
   Brief summary:

   ____

   ____

6. Abdominal scan
   ☐ Observed
   ☐ Assisted
   Brief summary:

   ____

   ____

7. Bio-development profile
   ☐ Observed
   ☐ Assisted
   Brief summary:

   ____

   ____

8. Fetal composition
   ☐ Observed
   ☐ Assisted
   Brief summary:

   ____

   ____

9. Amniocentesis
   ☐ Observed
   ☐ Assisted
   Brief summary:

   ____

   ____

(Continued)

Name ____

Plain Radiography

10. Chest
    - ☐ Observed
    - ☐ Assisted

    Brief summary:

    ____

    ____

11. Extremity
    - ☐ Observed
    - ☐ Assisted

    Brief summary:

    ____

    ____

12. Neck
    - ☐ Observed
    - ☐ Assisted

    Brief summary:

    ____

    ____

13. Ribs
    - ☐ Observed
    - ☐ Assisted

    Brief summary:

    ____

    ____

14. Spine
    - ☐ Observed
    - ☐ Assisted

    Brief summary:

    ____

    ____

15. KUB
    - ☐ Observed
    - ☐ Assisted

    Brief summary:

    ____

    ____

(Continued)

CT Scanning

16. Without contrast

☐ Observed

☐ Assisted

Brief summary:

____

____

17. With contrast

☐ Observed

☐ Assisted

Brief summary:

____

____

MRI

18. Head

☐ Observed

☐ Assisted

Brief summary:

____

____

19. Extremity

☐ Observed

☐ Assisted

Brief summary:

____

____

Nuclear Medicine

20. Cardiac stress test

☐ Observed

☐ Assisted

Brief summary:

____

____

(Continued)

Name ______________________________

21. Liver scan
    - ☐ Observed
    - ☐ Assisted

    Brief summary:

    ____

    ____

22. Spleen scan
    - ☐ Observed
    - ☐ Assisted

    Brief summary:

    ____

    ____

23. Bone scan
    - ☐ Observed
    - ☐ Assisted

    Brief summary:

    ____

    ____

Breast

24. Mammogram
    - ☐ Observed
    - ☐ Assisted

    Brief summary:

    ____

    ____

Endoscopy Procedures

25. Esophagogastroduodenoscopy
    - ☐ Observed
    - ☐ Assisted

    Brief summary:

    ____

    ____

26. Bronchoscopy
    - ☐ Observed
    - ☐ Assisted

    Brief summary:

    ____

    ____

(Continued)

27. Flexible sigmoidoscopy
   - ☐ Observed
   - ☐ Assisted

   Brief summary:

   ____

   ____

28. Capsule enteroscopy
   - ☐ Observed
   - ☐ Assisted

   Brief summary:

   ____

   ____

29. Fluoroscopy
   - ☐ Observed
   - ☐ Assisted

   Brief summary:

   ____

   ____

30. Gastroscopy
   - ☐ Observed
   - ☐ Assisted

   Brief summary:

   ____

   ____

31. Proctoscopy
   - ☐ Observed
   - ☐ Assisted

   Brief summary:

   ____

   ____

32. Biopsy
   - ☐ Observed
   - ☐ Assisted

   Brief summary:

   ____

   ____

(Continued)

Name ______________________________

33. Barium GI
    ☐ Observed
    ☐ Assisted
    Brief summary:

    ____

    ____

Equipment Usage

34. Scopes
    ☐ Observed
    ☐ Assisted
    Brief summary:

    ____

    ____

35. Pulse oximeter
    ☐ Observed
    ☐ Assisted
    Brief summary:

    ____

    ____

36. ECG monitor
    ☐ Observed
    ☐ Assisted
    Brief summary:

    ____

    ____

Client Care

37. Positioning
    ☐ Observed
    ☐ Assisted
    Brief summary:

    ____

    ____

38. Client anesthesia
    ☐ Observed
    ☐ Assisted
    Brief summary:

    ____

    ____

(Continued)

39. Dressing/Undressing
    ☐ Observed
    ☐ Assisted
    Brief summary:

    ____

    ____

Aseptic Procedures

40. Clean scopes, instruments
    ☐ Observed
    ☐ Assisted
    Brief summary:

    ____

    ____

41. Clean stretchers, carts
    ☐ Observed
    ☐ Assisted
    Brief summary:

    ____

    ____

42. Specimen collection
    ☐ Observed
    ☐ Assisted
    Brief summary:

    ____

    ____

43. Standard precautions
    ☐ Observed
    ☐ Assisted
    Brief summary:

    ____

    ____

44. Sterilization
    ☐ Observed
    ☐ Assisted
    Brief summary:

    ____

    ____

(Continued)

Name ____

Other

45. Transporting clients

    ☐ Observed

    ☐ Assisted

    Brief summary:

    ____

    ____

46. Client education/dismissal

    ☐ Observed

    ☐ Assisted

    Brief summary:

    ____

    ____

Student Name: ______________________________________

Technician Name: ___________________________________

Notes

Student ____________________ Dates __________ Site __________ Preceptor __________

Radiology Services Post-Clinical Reflection

Rotation Report

Overview

Instructions: Answer the following questions using complete sentences.

1. What were your responsibilities or duties this week?

____

____

2. What new knowledge or skill did you learn or observe this week?

____

____

3. What was the best thing that happened at your clinical site this week?

____

____

4. What was the most challenging thing that happened at your clinical site this week?

____

____

5. What problems or difficulties did you encounter or observe at your clinical site? How were they dealt with?

____

____

6. Was this week good, fair, or bad? Explain.

____

____

Observations

Instructions: List the observations you made for each of the following categories.

1. Technology observed:

____

____

2. Diagnostic procedures observed:

____

____

(Continued)

3. Therapeutic procedures observed:

____

____

4. Diseases or disorders observed:

____

____

5. Medical terminology or abbreviations encountered:

____

____

6. Other observations:

____

____

Supervisor Signature: ____________________

Date: ____________________

Rotation Journal

Instructions: Write a journal entry detailing your learning experience at the clinical rotation. Use the following topics to help write a complete journal entry.

Assessment of the Environment

- Personnel
- Services provided
- Equipment
- Technology utilized

Observation

- Health care providers
- Team skills
- Communication skills
- Safety procedures
- Therapeutic/diagnostic procedures

Knowledge

- New information learned
- Medical terminology
- Skills learned

Evaluation

- Personal experience
- Educational value
- Professional value

Journal Entry

Write a journal entry summarizing your clinical experience.

____

____

____

____

____

____

Name ______________________ Date ____________ Period ____________

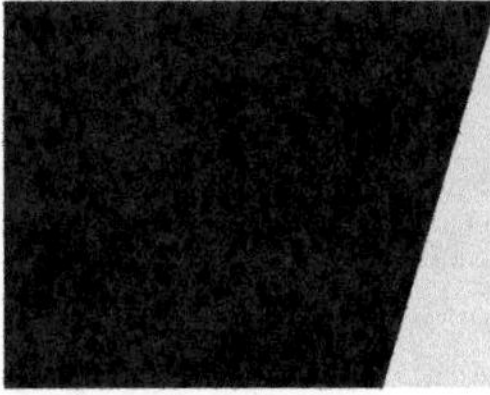

Rehabilitation Pre-Clinical Worksheet

Instructions: Answer the following questions.

1. Define the following terms.

   A. Edema:

   B. Atrophy:

   C. Contracture:

   D. Ataxia:

   E. Convulsion:

   F. Dystaxia:

   G. Hemiparesis:

   H. Hypertrophy:

   I. Hypotonia:

   J. Myalgia:

(Continued)

K. Myocele:

L. Myolysis:

M. Myoma:

N. Myorrhexis:

O. Rigor:

2. Three factors make the muscular system capable of moving the body: muscle type, muscle excitability and opposition between muscle pairs. Describe what is happening with each factor.
   A. Muscle type:

   B. Muscle excitability:

   C. Opposition between muscle pairs:

3. Describe how hemiplegia differs from paraplegia.

4. What is muscular dystrophy?

5. Differentiate between passive, active, and resistive ROM exercise.

(Continued)

Name ___________________________________

6. Define the following ROM terms.
   A. Abduction:
   B. Adduction:
   C. Flexion:
   D. Extension:
   E. Circumduction:
   F. Rotation:
   G. Pronation:
   H. Supination:
   I. Inversion:
   J. Eversion:
7. What are ADLs?
8. Define *adaptive equipment*.

(Continued)

9. Give three examples of adaptive equipment and what they are used for.

10. Describe the different types of joints in the body and give an example of each.

11. Differentiate between a sprain, a strain, and a dislocation.

12. Differentiate between fascia, a tendon, and a ligament.

13. Differentiate between rheumatoid arthritis and osteoarthritis.

14. What is gout?

15. What is rickets?

16. Describe the following types of treatments work.
   A. Arthroscopy:

   B. Hot pack:

   C. Cryotherapy:

   D. Brace:

(Continued)

Name ____

E. TENS unit/electrotherapy:

____

____

F. Ultrasound:

____

____

G. Acupuncture:

____

____

H. Hydrotherapy:

____

____

I. Wound therapy:

____

____

J. Aerobic therapy:

____

____

17. What is a prosthesis?

____

____

18. Describe the difference between physical therapy, occupational therapy, and kinesiology.

____

____

19. What are the five domains of therapeutic recreation?

____

____

20. What are the main goals of recreational therapy?

____

____

21. Describe the following types of recreational therapy:

A. Art and crafts:

____

____

(Continued)

B. Music:

C. Play therapy:

D. Pet therapy:

E. Sport therapy:

F. Drama:

G. Games:

H. Cooking:

22. The following activities are used in recreational therapy. Describe how each activity helps in the physical, social, and cognitive domains.
    A. Music therapy and a 72-year-old recovering from a stroke:

    B. Drama therapy and a 16-year-old recovery from a MVA resulting in death of best friend and amputation of right leg below the knee:

    C. Playing a video game with a 27-year-old who has muscular dystrophy and is wheelchair bound:

    D. Pet therapy for a 62-year-old experiencing early-stage Alzheimer's:

Name ______________________ Date ____________ Period ____________

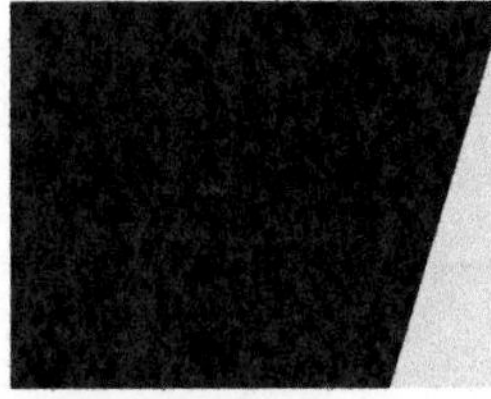

Rehabilitation Workplace Discovery Sheet

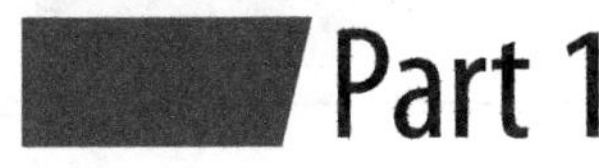

Part 1

During the Clinical Experience

Instructions: Answer the following questions.

1. Research the following diagnostic exams.
   A. Biopsy:

   ____

   ____

   B. Deep tendon reflexes:

   ____

   ____

   C. CT scan:

   ____

   ____

   D. Electromyogram:

   ____

   ____

   E. Goniometry:

   ____

   ____

   F. MRI:

   ____

   ____

   G. Nuclear medicine imaging:

   ____

   ____

   H. Radiography:

   ____

   ____

(Continued)

I. ROM:

____

____

J. Sonography:

____

____

2. Give three disorders or conditions a therapist would use the following therapies to treat.

A. Hot pack:

____

____

B. Cryotherapy:

____

____

C. Brace:

____

____

D. TENS unit/Electrotherapy:

____

____

E. Ultrasound:

____

____

F. Acupuncture:

____

____

G. Hydrotherapy:

____

____

H. Wound therapy:

____

____

3. You are a twenty-nine-year-old computer programmer with carpal tunnel syndrome. Research different kinds of treatments available.

____

____

(Continued)

Name ______________________________

4. How do you become a recreational therapist?

5. What type of facilities hire a recreational therapist?

6. How much of your time is spent one-on-one with a client?

7. How much of your time is spent doing group activities?

8. How much of your time is spent documenting?

9. List three activities that work well to help clients who need to work on fine motor skills.

10. List three activities that work well to help clients who need to work on social skills.

11. List four activities that help clients who need to work on memory.

12. List four activities that work well to help clients who need to work on gross motor skills.

(Continued)

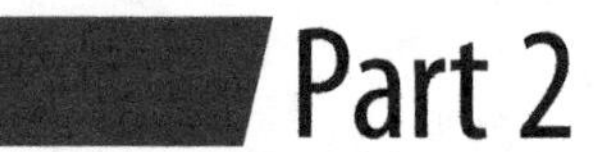

Part 2

After the Clinical Experience

Instructions: For each item below, identify whether you observed or assisted. Then, provide a brief summary.

Orientation

1. Rehabilitation services
   - ☐ Observed
   - ☐ Assisted

   Brief summary:

   ____

   ____

2. Recreational therapy
   - ☐ Observed
   - ☐ Assisted

   Brief summary:

   ____

   ____

Client Evaluation/Assessment

3. Musculoskeletal/Neurological
   - ☐ Observed
   - ☐ Assisted

   Brief summary:

   ____

   ____

4. Mobility/ambulation/range of motion
   - ☐ Observed
   - ☐ Assisted

   Brief summary:

   ____

   ____

5. Client teaching
   - ☐ Observed
   - ☐ Assisted

   Brief summary:

   ____

   ____

(Continued)

Name ____________________

Physical Therapy Treatment Modalities

6. Traction
   - ☐ Observed
   - ☐ Assisted

   Brief summary:

   ____

   ____

7. Hot packs/cryotherapy
   - ☐ Observed
   - ☐ Assisted

   Brief summary:

   ____

   ____

8. Ultrasound
   - ☐ Observed
   - ☐ Assisted

   Brief summary:

   ____

   ____

9. Massage
   - ☐ Observed
   - ☐ Assisted

   Brief summary:

   ____

   ____

10. Electrical stimulation
    - ☐ Observed
    - ☐ Assisted

    Brief summary:

    ____

    ____

11. Hydrotherapy
    - ☐ Observed
    - ☐ Assisted

    Brief summary:

    ____

    ____

(Continued)

Occupational Therapy Treatment Modalities

12. Paraffin bath

    ☐ Observed

    ☐ Assisted

    Brief summary:

    ____

    ____

13. TENS

    ☐ Observed

    ☐ Assisted

    Brief summary:

    ____

    ____

14. Splinting

    ☐ Observed

    ☐ Assisted

    Brief summary:

    ____

    ____

15. Infant stimulation

    ☐ Observed

    ☐ Assisted

    Brief summary:

    ____

    ____

16. Gait training with crutches/walker/cane

    ☐ Observed

    ☐ Assisted

    Brief summary:

    ____

    ____

Therapeutic Exercises

17. Strengthening/Coordination

    ☐ Observed

    ☐ Assisted

    Brief summary:

    ____

    ____

(Continued)

Name ______________________________

18. ADL

☐ Observed

☐ Assisted

Brief summary:

____

____

19. Endurance/Coordination

☐ Observed

☐ Assisted

Brief summary:

____

____

20. Stretching

☐ Observed

☐ Assisted

Brief summary:

____

____

Recreational Therapy

21. Develop and post activities on calendar

☐ Observed

☐ Assisted

Brief summary:

____

____

22. Make posters/mobiles/newsletters for individual activities

☐ Observed

☐ Assisted

Brief summary:

____

____

23. Assist clients to and from activities sessions

☐ Observed

☐ Assisted

Brief summary:

____

____

(Continued)

24. Encourage clients to participate in activities

☐ Observed

☐ Assisted

Brief summary:

____

____

25. Lead activity sessions

☐ Observed

☐ Assisted

Brief summary:

____

____

26. Interact with uninvolved clients

☐ Observed

☐ Assisted

Brief summary:

____

____

27. Integrate music therapy into activities

☐ Observed

☐ Assisted

Brief summary:

____

____

28. Distribute activity calendars and newsletters

☐ Observed

☐ Assisted

Brief summary:

____

____

29. Distribute mail to clients

☐ Observed

☐ Assisted

Brief summary:

____

____

(Continued)

Name ____

30. Assist in reading mail to clients
    - ☐ Observed
    - ☐ Assisted

    Brief summary:

    ____

    ____

31. Prepare mail for clients
    - ☐ Observed
    - ☐ Assisted

    Brief summary:

    ____

    ____

Student Name: ______________________________

Technician Name: ____________________________

Notes

Student ______________________ Dates ____________ Site ____________ Preceptor ____________

Rehabilitation Post-Clinical Reflection

Rotation Report

Overview

Instructions: Answer the following questions using complete sentences.

1. What were your responsibilities or duties this week?

____

____

2. What new knowledge or skill did you learn or observe this week?

____

____

3. What was the best thing that happened at your clinical site this week?

____

____

4. What was the most challenging thing that happened at your clinical site this week?

____

____

5. What problems or difficulties did you encounter or observe at your clinical site? How were they dealt with?

____

____

6. Was this week good, fair, or bad? Explain.

____

____

Observations

Instructions: List the observations you made for each of the following categories.

1. Technology observed:

____

____

2. Diagnostic procedures observed:

____

____

(Continued)

3. Therapeutic procedures observed:

____

____

4. Diseases or disorders observed:

____

____

5. Medical terminology or abbreviations encountered:

____

____

6. Other observations:

____

____

Supervisor Signature: ____________________

Date: ____________________

Rotation Journal

Instructions: Write a journal entry detailing your learning experience at the clinical rotation. Use the following topics to help write a complete journal entry.

Assessment of the Environment

- Personnel
- Services provided
- Equipment
- Technology utilized

Observation

- Health care providers
- Team skills
- Communication skills
- Safety procedures
- Therapeutic/diagnostic procedures

Knowledge

- New information learned
- Medical terminology
- Skills learned

Evaluation

- Personal experience
- Educational value
- Professional value

Journal Entry

Write a journal entry summarizing your clinical experience.

____

____

____

____

____

____

Name ______________________ Date ____________ Period ________

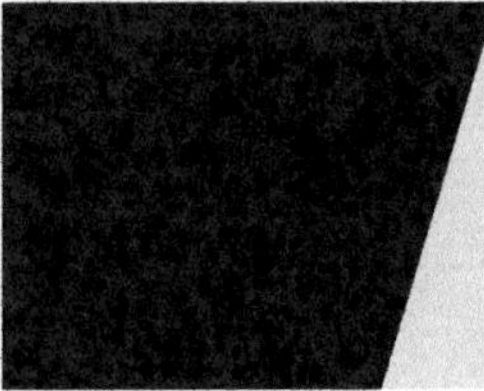

Reproductive Health Pre-Clinical Worksheet

Instructions: Answer the following questions.

1. Define the following terms related to obstetrics and gynecology.

   A. Antepartum:

   ____

   ____

   B. Braxton-Hicks contractions:

   ____

   ____

   C. Episiotomy:

   ____

   ____

   D. Family planning:

   ____

   ____

   E. Fundal height:

   ____

   ____

   F. Gestation:

   ____

   ____

   G. Gravida:

   ____

   ____

   H. Gynecology:

   ____

   ____

   I. Intrapartum:

   ____

   ____

   J. Mammogram:

   ____

   ____

(Continued)

K. Mastitis:

L. Obstetrics:

M. PAP smear:

N. Para:

O. Postpartum depression:

P. Postpartum:

2. What routine tests do all people who are pregnant receive?

3. What is prenatal care? Why is it important?

4. What is a normal fetal heart rate (FHR)?

5. Name and describe the stages and phases of labor:

A. Stage 1:

i. Stage 1 Phase 1:

ii. Stage 1 Phase 2:

iii. Stage 1 Phase 3:

(Continued)

B. Stage 2:
   i. Stage 2 Phase 1:

   ____

   ii. Stage 2 Phase 2:

   ____

   iii. Stage 2 Phase 3:

   ____

C. Stage 3:
   i. Stage 3 Phase 1:

   ____

   ii. Stage 3 Phase 2:

   ____

   iii. Stage 3 Phase 3:

   ____

D. Stage 4:
   i. Stage 4 Phase 1:

   ____

   ii. Stage 4 Phase 2:

   ____

   iii. Stage 4 Phase 3:

   ____

4. Describe the difference between cervical effacement and cervical dilation.

____

____

5. Define the following terms related to pregnancy and childbirth.

A. Acceleration:

____

____

B. AROM:

____

____

C. BOW:

____

____

D. C/S:

____

____

(Continued)

E. Crowning:

F. Deceleration:

G. FHR:

H. Nuchal cord:

I. OA:

J. OP:

K. Placenta previa:

L. Placental abruption:

M. Presenting part:

N. Prolapsed cord:

O. ROM:

P. SVD:

(Continued)

Q. Vertex:

____

____

6. What impact might the nuchal cord have on the fetus during the birthing process?

____

____

7. Explain the purpose of fundus checks.

____

____

8. What is the purpose of a sitz bath?

____

____

9. What is the treatment for mastitis?

____

____

10. Define and describe thrombophlebitis.

____

____

11. What is a puerperal infection?

____

____

12. List the normal ranges for vital signs in a newborn.

A. Temperature:

____

B. Pulse:

____

C. Respirations:

____

D. Blood pressure:

____

13. How often does the average baby have a bowel movement and void?

____

____

14. What is an APGAR? Explain the APGAR scoring of the newborn, including the normal values.

____

____

(Continued)

15. What routine procedures are performed on the newborn?

____

____

16. List the components of the newborn assessment. What reflexes are checked?

____

____

17. What security measures are used to keep newborns safe?

____

____

Name ______________________ Date ____________ Period __________

Reproductive Health Workplace Discovery Sheet

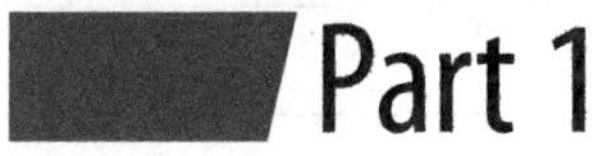

Part 1

During the Clinical Experience

Instructions: Answer the following questions.

1. What is the health care provider's title and program of study/major?

2. What is the health care provider's job description?

3. What educational training is required for this job?

4. What additional courses do you wish you had taken in high school or college to be more prepared for this field of work?

5. What do you like most about this career?

6. What do you dislike the most about this field?

7. How many clients do you see on a daily basis?

8. What other careers are associated with the employees that work in this office?

(Continued)

9. What type of equipment in this department looks familiar to you? (List at least three)

____

____

10. What type of equipment is specific to this care area? (List at least three)

____

____

Part 2

After the Clinical Experience

Instructions: For each item below, identify whether you observed or assisted. Then, provide a brief summary.

Client Services

1. Family planning
   ☐ Observed
   ☐ Assisted
   Brief summary:

   ____

   ____

2. Prenatal health
   ☐ Observed
   ☐ Assisted
   Brief summary:

   ____

   ____

3. Women's health
   ☐ Observed
   ☐ Assisted
   Brief summary:

   ____

   ____

4. Emergency procedures
   ☐ Observed
   ☐ Assisted
   Brief summary:

   ____

   ____

(Continued)

Name ____________________________

Health Promotion

5. Identification of health issues

☐ Observed

☐ Assisted

Brief summary:

____

____

6. Disease prevention

☐ Observed

☐ Assisted

Brief summary:

____

____

Routine Care

7. Antepartum

☐ Observed

☐ Assisted

Brief summary:

____

____

8. Intrapartum

☐ Observed

☐ Assisted

Brief summary:

____

____

9. Postpartum

☐ Observed

☐ Assisted

Brief summary:

____

____

(Continued)

Admission Processing

10. Triage

    ☐ Observed

    ☐ Assisted

    Brief summary:

    ____

    ____

11. Observation vs admission

    ☐ Observed

    ☐ Assisted

    Brief summary:

    ____

    ____

12. Assembling records

    ☐ Observed

    ☐ Assisted

    Brief summary:

    ____

    ____

13. Consents

    ☐ Observed

    ☐ Assisted

    Brief summary:

    ____

    ____

14. Confidentiality

    ☐ Observed

    ☐ Assisted

    Brief summary:

    ____

    ____

15. Provider notification

    ☐ Observed

    ☐ Assisted

    Brief summary:

    ____

    ____

(Continued)

Name ______________________________

16. Intake and output
    - ☐ Observed
    - ☐ Assisted

    Brief summary:

    ____

    ____

17. Setting up a room
    - ☐ Observed
    - ☐ Assisted

    Brief summary:

    ____

    ____

Labor Process

18. Stages of labor
    - ☐ Observed
    - ☐ Assisted

    Brief summary:

    ____

    ____

19. Fetal monitoring
    - ☐ Observed
    - ☐ Assisted

    Brief summary:

    ____

    ____

20. Client management and labor support
    - ☐ Observed
    - ☐ Assisted

    Brief summary:

    ____

    ____

21. Obtaining vital signs
    - ☐ Observed
    - ☐ Assisted

    Brief summary:

    ____

    ____

(Continued)

22. Pain management
   ☐ Observed
   ☐ Assisted
   Brief summary:

   ____

   ____

23. Potential complications
   ☐ Observed
   ☐ Assisted
   Brief summary:

   ____

   ____

24. Cesarean deliveries
   ☐ Observed
   ☐ Assisted
   Brief summary:

   ____

   ____

Recovery

25. Bleeding management
   ☐ Observed
   ☐ Assisted
   Brief summary:

   ____

   ____

26. Fundal checks
   ☐ Observed
   ☐ Assisted
   Brief summary:

   ____

   ____

27. Skin-to-skin
   ☐ Observed
   ☐ Assisted
   Brief summary:

   ____

   ____

(Continued)

Name ___________________________________

28. Infant feeding assistance
    ☐ Observed
    ☐ Assisted
    Brief summary:
    ____
    ____

29. Transfer to mother-baby
    ☐ Observed
    ☐ Assisted
    Brief summary:
    ____
    ____

30. Vital signs on mother
    ☐ Observed
    ☐ Assisted
    Brief summary:
    ____
    ____

31. Ambulating client
    ☐ Observed
    ☐ Assisted
    Brief summary:
    ____
    ____

32. Giving client a shower
    ☐ Observed
    ☐ Assisted
    Brief summary:
    ____
    ____

33. Make client's bed
    ☐ Observed
    ☐ Assisted
    Brief summary:
    ____
    ____

(Continued)

34. Clean client's room
   ☐ Observed
   ☐ Assisted
   Brief summary:

   ____

   ____

35. Empty urinary drainage system
   ☐ Observed
   ☐ Assisted
   Brief summary:

   ____

   ____

36. Obtain client's daily weight
   ☐ Observed
   ☐ Assisted
   Brief summary:

   ____

   ____

Infant care

37. APGAR scores
   ☐ Observed
   ☐ Assisted
   Brief summary:

   ____

   ____

38. Newborn assessment
   ☐ Observed
   ☐ Assisted
   Brief summary:

   ____

   ____

39. Routine care
   ☐ Observed
   ☐ Assisted
   Brief summary:

   ____

   ____

(Continued)

Name ______________________________

40. Hearing screening on baby

☐ Observed

☐ Assisted

Brief summary:

____

____

41. Giving baby a bath

☐ Observed

☐ Assisted

Brief summary:

____

____

42. Medications

☐ Observed

☐ Assisted

Brief summary:

____

____

43. Immunizations for baby

☐ Observed

☐ Assisted

Brief summary:

____

____

44. Circumcision

☐ Observed

☐ Assisted

Brief summary:

____

____

45. Newborn complications

☐ Observed

☐ Assisted

Brief summary:

____

____

(Continued)

Communication

46. Oral
    - ☐ Observed
    - ☐ Assisted

    Brief summary:

    ____

    ____

47. Written
    - ☐ Observed
    - ☐ Assisted

    Brief summary:

    ____

    ____

48. Record keeping
    - ☐ Observed
    - ☐ Assisted

    Brief summary:

    ____

    ____

Student Name: ______________________________

Technician Name: ______________________________

Student ______________________ Dates ____________ Site ____________ Preceptor ____________

Reproductive Health Post-Clinical Reflection

Rotation Report

Overview

Instructions: Answer the following questions using complete sentences.

1. What were your responsibilities or duties this week?

____

____

2. What new knowledge or skill did you learn or observe this week?

____

____

3. What was the best thing that happened at your clinical site this week?

____

____

4. What was the most challenging thing that happened at your clinical site this week?

____

____

5. What problems or difficulties did you encounter or observe at your clinical site? How were they dealt with?

____

____

6. Was this week good, fair, or bad? Explain.

____

____

Observations

Instructions: List the observations you made for each of the following categories.

1. Technology observed:

____

____

2. Diagnostic procedures observed:

____

____

(Continued)

3. Therapeutic procedures observed:

____

____

4. Diseases or disorders observed:

____

____

5. Medical terminology or abbreviations encountered:

____

____

6. Other observations:

____

____

Supervisor Signature: ______________________________

Date: ______________________________

Rotation Journal

Instructions: Write a journal entry detailing your learning experience at the clinical rotation. Use the following topics to help write a complete journal entry.

Assessment of the Environment

- Personnel
- Services provided
- Equipment
- Technology utilized

Observation

- Health care providers
- Team skills
- Communication skills
- Safety procedures
- Therapeutic/diagnostic procedures

Knowledge

- New information learned
- Medical terminology
- Skills learned

Evaluation

- Personal experience
- Educational value
- Professional value

Journal Entry

Write a journal entry summarizing your clinical experience.

____

____

____

____

____

____

Name ______________________ Date ____________ Period ____________

Skeletomuscular Pre-Clinical Worksheet

Instructions: Answer the following questions.

1. What is a chiropractic adjustment? What is the goal of a chiropractic adjustment?

2. What are the neurological, vascular, and respiratory benefits of chiropractic care?

3. What are the risks of chiropractic cervical adjustments?

4. Are any tools used to perform chiropractic adjustments? If so, what are they?

5. What types of clients may require special adjustments or may be difficult to adjust?

6. What types of health issues are typically treated by chiropractors?

7. What other types of treatments might a chiropractor use in addition to adjustments?

8. Define the following terms related to chiropractic.
   A. Subluxation:

   B. Cavitation:

   C. Dynamic thrust:

(Continued)

D. Intervertebral disk:

____

____

9. Label the following diagram with the correct anatomical terms:

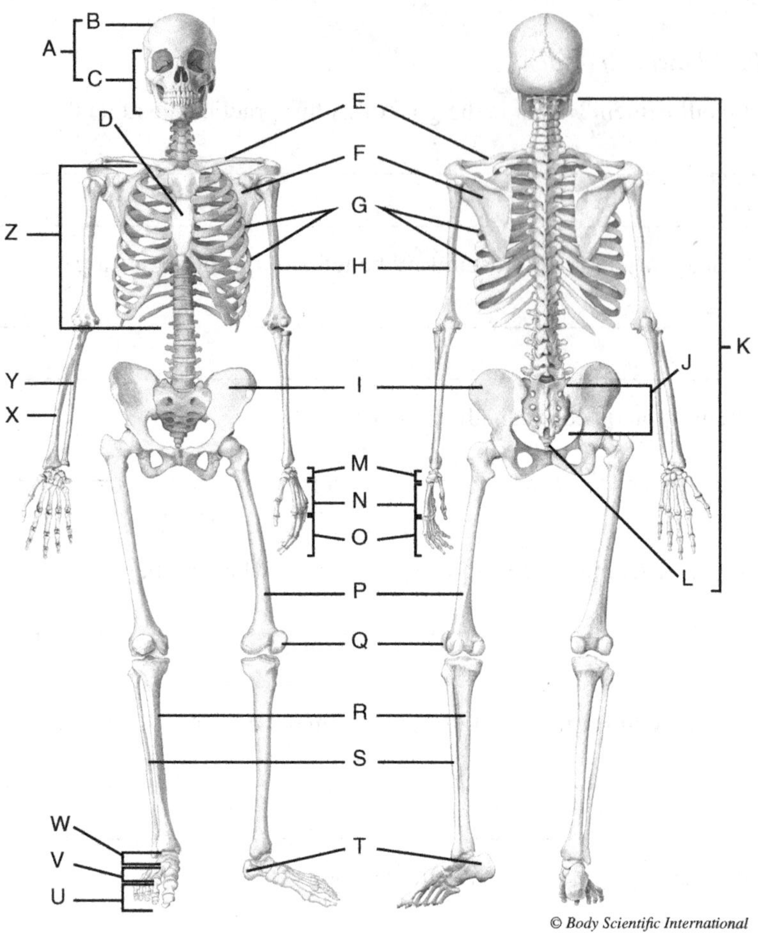

A. ______________________ N. ______________________

B. ______________________ O. ______________________

C. ______________________ P. ______________________

D. ______________________ Q. ______________________

E. ______________________ R. ______________________

F. ______________________ S. ______________________

G. ______________________ T. ______________________

H. ______________________ U. ______________________

I. ______________________ V. ______________________

J. ______________________ W. ______________________

K. ______________________ X. ______________________

L. ______________________ Y. ______________________

M. ______________________ Z. ______________________

(Continued)

Name ______________________________

10. Define the following skeletal terms:

A. Diaphysis:

____

____

B. Epiphysis:

____

____

C. Sesamoid bone:

____

____

D. Bone process:

____

____

E. Bone depression:

____

____

11. Define the following directional terms:

A. Superior:

____

____

B. Inferior:

____

____

C. Cranial:

____

____

D. Caudal:

____

____

E. Ventral:

____

____

F. Dorsal:

____

____

(Continued)

G. Medial:

____

____

H. Lateral:

____

____

I. Proximal:

____

____

J. Distal:

____

____

12. Briefly describe the following skeletal procedures and treatments:

A. Arthroscopy:

____

____

B. Myelogram:

____

____

C. Closed reduction:

____

____

D. Open reduction:

____

____

E. Diskectomy:

____

____

F. Arthrocentesis:

____

____

G. Arthrodesis:

____

____

H. Osteotomy:

____

____

(Continued)

Name ______________________________

I. Synovectomy:

J. Minimally invasive TJR:

K. Splint:

L. Brace:

M. Cast:

N. Traction:

O. Physical therapy:

13. Describe the following types of fractures:

A. Comminuted:

B. Compound:

C. Greenstick:

D. Longitudinal:

E. Oblique:

(Continued)

F. Pathological:

G. Simple fracture:

H. Spiral fracture:

I. Transverse:

J. Compressor fracture of the back:

14. Describe the following skeletal disorders/diseases:

A. Dislocation:

B. Sprain:

C. Strain:

D. Compartment syndrome:

E. Amputations:

F. Arthritis:

G. Bursitis:

(Continued)

Name ____________________

H. Chondromalacia:

____

____

I. Fracture:

____

____

J. Osteomalacia:

____

____

K. Osteopenia:

____

____

L. Osteoporosis:

____

____

M. Subluxation:

____

____

N. Tendinitis:

____

____

15. Differentiate between an MRI, CAT/CT scan, and normal X-ray.

____

____

Notes

Name ______________________________ Date ______________ Period ____________

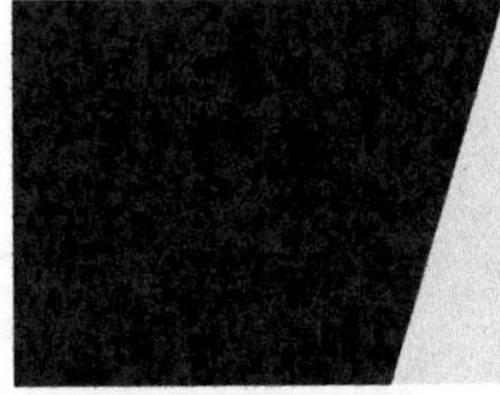

Skeletomuscular Workplace Discovery Sheet

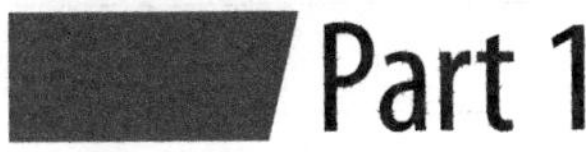

Part 1

During the Clinical Experience

Instructions: Answer the following questions.

1. What is your title and what was your program of study/major?

____

____

2. What is your job description?

____

____

3. What educational training is required for this job?

____

____

4. What additional courses do you wish you had taken in high school or college to be more prepared for this field of work?

____

____

5. What do you like most about this career?

____

____

6. What do you dislike the most about this field?

____

____

7. How many clients do you see on a daily basis?

____

____

8. What other careers are associated with the employees that work in this office?

____

____

(Continued)

9. What is the most common type of orthopedic surgery procedure seen in this unit?

10. What is the goal for getting a client up and moving after surgery?

11. When do most clients begin PT and/or OT after surgery?

12. What are the criteria for releasing clients from the PACU to the floor?

13. What are the criteria for dismissing the client?

14. What client education is done at dismissal?

15. For clients who need assistive devices, such as CPM machines or walkers, do most clients take them home or do they purchase them outside of the hospital?

16. What type of equipment in this department looks familiar to you? (List at least three.)

17. What type of equipment is specific to this care area? (List at least three.)

(Continued)

Name ____

Part 2

After the Clinical Experience

Instructions: For each item below, identify whether you observed or assisted. Then, provide a brief summary.

Client Services

1. Client screening
   - ☐ Observed
   - ☐ Assisted

   Brief summary:

   ____

   ____

2. Client assessment
   - ☐ Observed
   - ☐ Assisted

   Brief summary:

   ____

   ____

3. Emergency procedures
   - ☐ Observed
   - ☐ Assisted

   Brief summary:

   ____

   ____

4. Scheduling procedures
   - ☐ Observed
   - ☐ Assisted

   Brief summary:

   ____

   ____

Health Promotion

5. Identification of health issues
   - ☐ Observed
   - ☐ Assisted

   Brief summary:

   ____

   ____

(Continued)

6. Disease prevention
   - ☐ Observed
   - ☐ Assisted

   Brief summary:

   ____

   ____

7. Impact of environmental factors
   - ☐ Observed
   - ☐ Assisted

   Brief summary:

   ____

   ____

Therapy Offered

8. Spinal decompression
   - ☐ Observed
   - ☐ Assisted

   Brief summary:

   ____

   ____

9. Acupuncture
   - ☐ Observed
   - ☐ Assisted

   Brief summary:

   ____

   ____

10. Myofascial release
    - ☐ Observed
    - ☐ Assisted

    Brief summary:

    ____

    ____

11. Trigger point therapy
    - ☐ Observed
    - ☐ Assisted

    Brief summary:

    ____

    ____

(Continued)

Name ____

Basic Client Care

12. Vital signs
    - ☐ Observed
    - ☐ Assisted

    Brief summary:

    ____

    ____

13. Intake and output
    - ☐ Observed
    - ☐ Assisted

    Brief summary:

    ____

    ____

14. Medication administration
    - ☐ Observed
    - ☐ Assisted

    Brief summary:

    ____

    ____

15. Epidural catheter
    - ☐ Observed
    - ☐ Assisted

    Brief summary:

    ____

    ____

16. IV pain management
    - ☐ Observed
    - ☐ Assisted

    Brief summary:

    ____

    ____

17. Meals/Nourishment
    - ☐ Observed
    - ☐ Assisted

    Brief summary:

    ____

    ____

(Continued)

18. Bathing/ADL
    ☐ Observed
    ☐ Assisted
    Brief summary:

    ____

    ____

Preoperative Client

19. Pre-op checklist
    ☐ Observed
    ☐ Assisted
    Brief summary:

    ____

    ____

20. Client assessment
    ☐ Observed
    ☐ Assisted
    Brief summary:

    ____

    ____

21. Client teaching
    ☐ Observed
    ☐ Assisted
    Brief summary:

    ____

    ____

Postoperative Client

22. Client monitoring
    ☐ Observed
    ☐ Assisted
    Brief summary:

    ____

    ____

23. Positioning/Early ambulation
    ☐ Observed
    ☐ Assisted
    Brief summary:

    ____

    ____

(Continued)

Name ____

24. Breathing and coughing
    - ☐ Observed
    - ☐ Assisted

    Brief summary:

    ____

    ____

25. Pain control
    - ☐ Observed
    - ☐ Assisted

    Brief summary:

    ____

    ____

26. TEDS antiembolism stockings
    - ☐ Observed
    - ☐ Assisted

    Brief summary:

    ____

    ____

27. Dressings/drains/hemovacs
    - ☐ Observed
    - ☐ Assisted

    Brief summary:

    ____

    ____

28. Pins, splints, casts
    - ☐ Observed
    - ☐ Assisted

    Brief summary:

    ____

    ____

Non-Surgical Client

29. Diagnostic tests
    - ☐ Observed
    - ☐ Assisted

    Brief summary:

    ____

    ____

(Continued)

30. Traction/Ambulation devices
   ☐ Observed
   ☐ Assisted
   Brief summary:

   ____

   ____

Communication

31. Oral
   ☐ Observed
   ☐ Assisted
   Brief summary:

   ____

   ____

32. Written
   ☐ Observed
   ☐ Assisted
   Brief summary:

   ____

   ____

33. Record keeping
   ☐ Observed
   ☐ Assisted
   Brief summary:

   ____

   ____

Student Name: ______________________________

Technician Name: ______________________________

Student ______________________ Dates ______________ Site ______________ Preceptor ______________

Skeletomuscular Post-Clinical Reflection

Rotation Report

Overview

Instructions: Answer the following questions using complete sentences.

1. What were your responsibilities or duties this week?

____

____

2. What new knowledge or skill did you learn or observe this week?

____

____

3. What was the best thing that happened at your clinical site this week?

____

____

4. What was the most challenging thing that happened at your clinical site this week?

____

____

5. What problems or difficulties did you encounter or observe at your clinical site? How were they dealt with?

____

____

6. Was this week good, fair, or bad? Explain.

____

____

Observations

Instructions: List the observations you made for each of the following categories.

1. Technology observed:

____

____

2. Diagnostic procedures observed:

____

____

(Continued)

3. Therapeutic procedures observed:

____

____

4. Diseases or disorders observed:

____

____

5. Medical terminology or abbreviations encountered:

____

____

6. Other observations:

____

____

Supervisor Signature: ______________________________

Date: ______________________________

Rotation Journal

Instructions: Write a journal entry detailing your learning experience at the clinical rotation. Use the following topics to help write a complete journal entry.

Assessment of the Environment

- Personnel
- Services provided
- Equipment
- Technology utilized

Observation

- Health care providers
- Team skills
- Communication skills
- Safety procedures
- Therapeutic/diagnostic procedures

Knowledge

- New information learned
- Medical terminology
- Skills learned

Evaluation

- Personal experience
- Educational value
- Professional value

Journal Entry

Write a journal entry summarizing your clinical experience.

____

____

____

____

____

____

Name ______________________ Date ______________ Period ____________

Surgery Pre-Clinical Worksheet

Instructions: Answer the following questions.

1. What must be included on a medical/surgical informed consent form?

____

____

2. Who can sign the medical/surgical consent form?

____

____

3. What is an advance directive?

____

____

4. Identify the five most common surgical procedures performed in day surgery.

____

____

5. Define the following terms related to surgery.

   A. Chest X-ray:

   ____

   ____

   B. EKG:

   ____

   ____

   C. CBC:

   ____

   ____

   D. UA:

   ____

   ____

   E. HCG:

   ____

   ____

   F. Coagulation studies:

   ____

   ____

(Continued)

G. Chem profile:

____

____

H. NPO:

____

____

I. NKDA:

____

____

J. Sterile field:

____

____

K. Neurological assessment:

____

____

6. Why is a pregnancy test run before day surgery?

____

____

7. What is a nosocomial infection?

____

____

8. What is anesthesia?

____

____

9. Describe five different types of anesthesia seen in a day surgery area.

____

____

10. Differentiate between intubation and extubating.

____

____

11. What is the PACU?

____

____

Name ______________________ Date ____________ Period ____________

Surgery Workplace Discovery Sheet

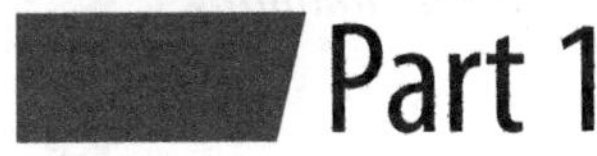

Part 1

During the Clinical Experience

Instructions: Answer the following questions.

1. What methods were used by the staff to verify the identity of the client during surgical rotation?

____

____

2. List the common forms required for admission to the day surgery unit.

____

____

3. What are the components of a client assessment in the pre-op area?

____

____

4. What client monitoring is performed during the recovery process?

____

____

5. What are three of the most common side effects of general anesthesia?

____

____

6. Identify the criteria for client discharge?

____

____

7. What are common topics covered by the staff with the client and client's family before discharge? List at least four.

____

____

(Continued)

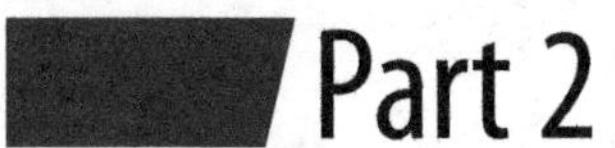

Part 2

After the Clinical Experience

Instructions: For each item below, identify whether you observed or assisted. Then, provide a brief summary.

Preoperative

1. Client admission
   ☐ Observed
   ☐ Assisted
   Brief summary:
   ____
   ____

2. Preoperative teaching
   ☐ Observed
   ☐ Assisted
   Brief summary:
   ____
   ____

3. Vital signs
   ☐ Observed
   ☐ Assisted
   Brief summary:
   ____
   ____

4. Starting IV
   ☐ Observed
   ☐ Assisted
   Brief summary:
   ____
   ____

5. Informed consent
   ☐ Observed
   ☐ Assisted
   Brief summary:
   ____
   ____

(Continued)

Name ____

Recovery

6. Client monitoring
   ☐ Observed
   ☐ Assisted
   Brief summary:
   ____
   ____

7. Vital signs
   ☐ Observed
   ☐ Assisted
   Brief summary:
   ____
   ____

8. Suctioning
   ☐ Observed
   ☐ Assisted
   Brief summary:
   ____
   ____

9. Extubating
   ☐ Observed
   ☐ Assisted
   Brief summary:
   ____
   ____

10. Operative site check
   ☐ Observed
   ☐ Assisted
   Brief summary:
   ____
   ____

11. Neurological assessment
   ☐ Observed
   ☐ Assisted
   Brief summary:
   ____
   ____

(Continued)

12. Post-anesthesia recovery
    ☐ Observed
    ☐ Assisted
    Brief summary:

    ____

    ____

13. Pain management
    ☐ Observed
    ☐ Assisted
    Brief summary:

    ____

    ____

Surgical Team

14. Members/Responsibilities
    ☐ Observed
    ☐ Assisted
    Brief summary:

    ____

    ____

15. Sterile/Nonsterile
    ☐ Observed
    ☐ Assisted
    Brief summary:

    ____

    ____

16. Client identification
    ☐ Observed
    ☐ Assisted
    Brief summary:

    ____

    ____

17. Care of surgical specimens
    ☐ Observed
    ☐ Assisted
    Brief summary:

    ____

    ____

(Continued)

Name ____

18. Identify basic surgical packs and instruments
    ☐ Observed
    ☐ Assisted
    Brief summary:
    ____
    ____

Aseptic Technique

19. Surgical scrub
    ☐ Observed
    ☐ Assisted
    Brief summary:
    ____
    ____

20. Gown and glove
    ☐ Observed
    ☐ Assisted
    Brief summary:
    ____
    ____

21. Sterile field
    ☐ Observed
    ☐ Assisted
    Brief summary:
    ____
    ____

22. Contaminated disposals
    ☐ Observed
    ☐ Assisted
    Brief summary:
    ____
    ____

Surgical Technique

23. Positioning
    ☐ Observed
    ☐ Assisted
    Brief summary:
    ____
    ____

(Continued)

24. Types of incisions
    ☐ Observed
    ☐ Assisted
    Brief summary:

    ____

    ____

25. Wound closure
    ☐ Observed
    ☐ Assisted
    Brief summary:

    ____

    ____

Anesthesiology

26. Types of anesthetics
    ☐ Observed
    ☐ Assisted
    Brief summary:

    ____

    ____

27. Types of induction
    ☐ Observed
    ☐ Assisted
    Brief summary:

    ____

    ____

28. Intubation
    ☐ Observed
    ☐ Assisted
    Brief summary:

    ____

    ____

Student Name: ______________________________

Technician Name: ____________________________

Student ______________________ Dates ____________ Site ____________ Preceptor ____________

Surgery Post-Clinical Reflection

Rotation Report

Overview

Instructions: Answer the following questions using complete sentences.

1. What were your responsibilities or duties this week?

____

____

2. What new knowledge or skill did you learn or observe this week?

____

____

3. What was the best thing that happened at your clinical site this week?

____

____

4. What was the most challenging thing that happened at your clinical site this week?

____

____

5. What problems or difficulties did you encounter or observe at your clinical site? How were they dealt with?

____

____

6. Was this week good, fair, or bad? Explain.

____

____

Observations

Instructions: List the observations you made for each of the following categories.

1. Technology observed:

____

____

2. Diagnostic procedures observed:

____

____

(Continued)

3. Therapeutic procedures observed:

____

____

4. Diseases or disorders observed:

____

____

5. Medical terminology or abbreviations encountered:

____

____

6. Other observations:

____

____

Supervisor Signature: ______________________________

Date: ______________________________

Rotation Journal

Instructions: Write a journal entry detailing your learning experience at the clinical rotation. Use the following topics to help write a complete journal entry.

Assessment of the Environment

- Personnel
- Services provided
- Equipment
- Technology utilized

Observation

- Health care providers
- Team skills
- Communication skills
- Safety procedures
- Therapeutic/diagnostic procedures

Knowledge

- New information learned
- Medical terminology
- Skills learned

Evaluation

- Personal experience
- Educational value
- Professional value

Journal Entry

Write a journal entry summarizing your clinical experience.

____

____

____

____

____

____

Name ______________________________ Date ______________ Period ____________

Urinary Pre-Clinical Worksheet

Instructions: Answer the following questions.

1. Label the part of the kidney.

   A. ______________________
   B. ______________________
   C. ______________________
   D. ______________________
   E. ______________________
   F. ______________________
   G. ______________________
   H. ______________________
   I. ______________________

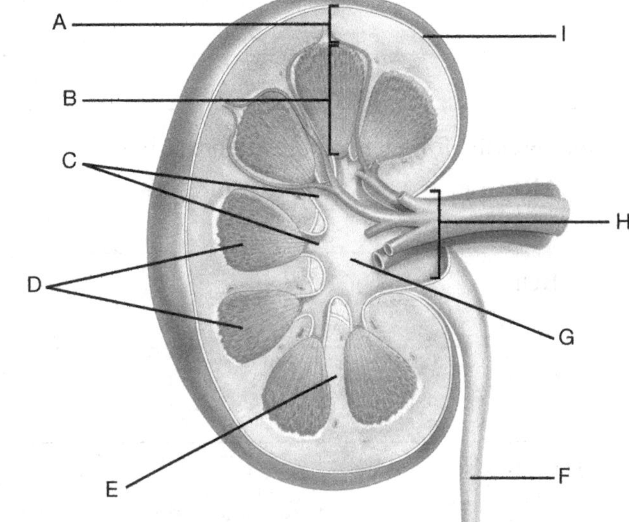

© Body Scientific International

2. The urinary system performs four major functions in the human body. Briefly describe what is happening in each of the following listed functions.

   A. Filtration:

   ____

   B. Waste storage and excretion:

   ____

   C. Hormone production:

   ____

   D. Homeostasis maintenance:

   ____

3. What types of shunts are used with dialysis clients and how do they differ from each other?

   ____

(Continued)

4. What is the difference between a straight catheter and a foley catheter?

5. What is a diuretic?

6. What are the lab tests BUN and creatinine measuring?

7. Interpret the following abbreviations.
   A. ARF:
   B. BUN:
   C. Cath:
   D. CRF:
   E. FF:
   F. GFR:
   G. I/O:
   H. IVP:
   I. KUB:
   J. PKD:
   K. PKU:
   L. SP GR:
   M. TNTC:
   N. UA:

(Continued)

Name ______________________________

O. UTI:

____

8. What is urology?

____

____

9. Label the following diagram of the urinary system.

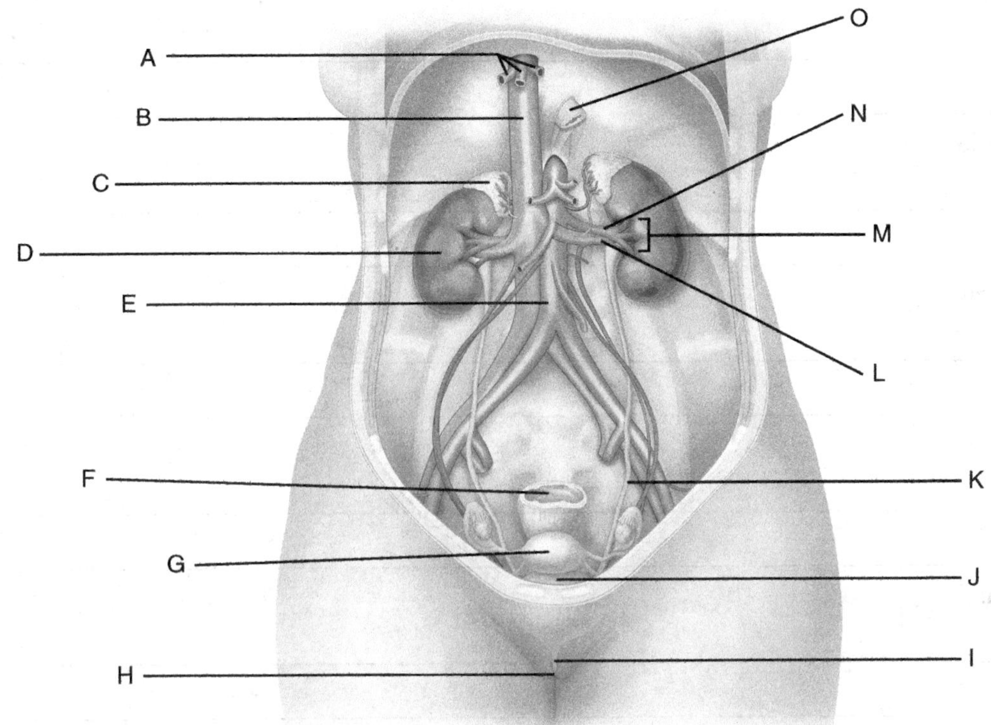

A. ______________ I. ______________

B. ______________ J. ______________

C. ______________ K. ______________

D. ______________ L. ______________

E. ______________ M. ______________

F. ______________ N. ______________

G. ______________ O. ______________

H. ______________

10. Define the following signs and symptoms.

A. Anuria:

____

____

(Continued)

B. Diuresis:

C. Dysuria:

D. Enuresis:

E. Glycosuria:

F. Hematuria:

G. Nocturnal enuresis:

H. Oliguria:

I. Polyuria:

J. Prolapse:

K. Urinary incontinence:

L. Urinary retention:

M. Urinary urgency:

(Continued)

Name ____________________

11. Describe the following diagnostic procedure.

A. Biopsy:

____

____

B. Cystoscope:

____

____

C. Gleason score (GS):

____

____

D. KUB:

____

____

E. BUN/Creatinine:

____

____

F. PSA:

____

____

G. Toxicology:

____

____

H. UA dipstick:

____

____

I. Specific gravity:

____

____

J. Sonography:

____

____

K. CT scan:

____

____

L. IVP:

____

____

(Continued)

M. Renal angiogram:

12. Compare and contrast the advantages and disadvantages of hemodialysis and peritoneal dialysis.

13. Define the following diseases/conditions as they pertain to the urinary system.

A. Cystitis:

B. Cystocele:

C. Cystolithiasis:

D. Diabetes:

E. Glomerulonephritis:

F. Nephrolithiasis:

G. Nephrosclerosis:

H. Polycystic kidney disease:

I. Pyelonephritis:

J. Renal cell carcinoma:

(Continued)

Name ______________________________

K. Renal failure:

L. Renal hypertension:

M. Renal ischemia:

N. Urinary tract infection (UTI):

O. Vesicovaginal fistula:

P. Wilms tumor:

14. Describe the following treatments.

A. Antibiotic:

B. Colposuspension:

C. Diuretic:

D. Lithotripsy:

E. Kidney transplant:

F. Lithotomy:

(Continued)

G. Nephrectomy:

____

____

H. Renal angioplasty:

____

____

I. Radical prostatectomy:

____

____

J. TURP:

____

____

K. Urinary catheterization:

____

____

L. Vasectomy:

____

____

Name ______________________ Date ____________ Period ____________

Urinary Workplace Discovery Sheet

Part 1

During the Clinical Experience

Instructions: Answer the following questions.

1. What kind of training is required to work in hemodialysis?

2. What is the difference between hemodialysis and peritoneal dialysis?

3. Do you work with patients who are to be released from the hospital and are planning on using peritoneal dialysis at home?

4. On average what percentage of patients choose hemodialysis over peritoneal dialysis?

5. What is the average length of each treatment, and how often do patients need to go through treatment?

6. What lab tests are run before and after treatment?

7. What side effects can occur from hemodialysis?

8. Describe the procedure for starting the patient on dialysis.

(Continued)

9. Will most of your patients require a kidney transplant at some point?

10. What patient education does your unit do?

11. Procedures such as vasectomy are done routinely in the office. Describe the procedure.

12. What patient education is given to patients before dismissing them to go home after a vasectomy?

13. What is the prognosis of a successful reversal of a vasectomy compared to reversal of a tubal ligation?

14. What are some of the common causes of UTIs in males?

15. What are some of the common causes of kidney stones in males?

16. What is the most common cause of benign prostatic hyperplasia?

Part 2

After the Clinical Experience

Instructions: For each item below, identify whether you observed or assisted. Then, provide a brief summary.

Routine Administrative Skills

1. Client record
   - ☐ Observed
   - ☐ Assisted

   Brief summary:

(Continued)

Name ____

2. Computerized record system
   ☐ Observed
   ☐ Assisted
   Brief summary:

   ____

   ____

Hemodialysis Procedures

3. Primary setup of dialysis machines
   ☐ Observed
   ☐ Assisted
   Brief summary:

   ____

   ____

4. Installation of filter
   ☐ Observed
   ☐ Assisted
   Brief summary:

   ____

   ____

5. Client connection to dialysis machine
   ☐ Observed
   ☐ Assisted
   Brief summary:

   ____

   ____

6. Disconnection of client from dialysis machine
   ☐ Observed
   ☐ Assisted
   Brief summary:

   ____

   ____

7. Post cleaning procedure of the dialysis machine
   ☐ Observed
   ☐ Assisted
   Brief summary:

   ____

   ____

(Continued)

Types of Shunts

8. Fistula arteriovenous graft

   ☐ Observed

   ☐ Assisted

   Brief summary:

   ____

   ____

9. Subclavian–Catheter Quinton

   ☐ Observed

   ☐ Assisted

   Brief summary:

   ____

   ____

10. Jugular–Catheter Quinton

    ☐ Observed

    ☐ Assisted

    Brief summary:

    ____

    ____

11. Permcath–Long-term temporary

    ☐ Observed

    ☐ Assisted

    Brief summary:

    ____

    ____

12. Femoral–Quinton or Permcath

    ☐ Observed

    ☐ Assisted

    Brief summary:

    ____

    ____

Urology Procedures

13. ESWL

    ☐ Observed

    ☐ Assisted

    Brief summary:

    ____

    ____

(Continued)

Name ____

14. Cystoscopy
    ☐ Observed
    ☐ Assisted
    Brief summary:

    ____

    ____

15. Ureteroscopy
    ☐ Observed
    ☐ Assisted
    Brief summary:

    ____

    ____

16. Stent placement
    ☐ Observed
    ☐ Assisted
    Brief summary:

    ____

    ____

17. Basket extraction
    ☐ Observed
    ☐ Assisted
    Brief summary:

    ____

    ____

18. TURP
    ☐ Observed
    ☐ Assisted
    Brief summary:

    ____

    ____

19. TURB
    ☐ Observed
    ☐ Assisted
    Brief summary:

    ____

    ____

(Continued)

20. KUB
☐ Observed
☐ Assisted
Brief summary:

____

____

21. Urinalysis
☐ Observed
☐ Assisted
Brief summary:

____

____

Patient Teaching

22. Preoperative
☐ Observed
☐ Assisted
Brief summary:

____

____

23. Postoperative
☐ Observed
☐ Assisted
Brief summary:

____

____

Clinical Signs and Symptoms

24. Psychological
☐ Observed
☐ Assisted
Brief summary:

____

____

25. Common diseases
☐ Observed
☐ Assisted
Brief summary:

____

____

(Continued)

Name ______________________________

Infection Control

26. Ultrasonic cleaning
    - ☐ Observed
    - ☐ Assisted

    Brief summary:

    ____

    ____

27. Sterile technique
    - ☐ Observed
    - ☐ Assisted

    Brief summary:

    ____

    ____

28. Isolation
    - ☐ Observed
    - ☐ Assisted

    Brief summary:

    ____

    ____

Laboratory

29. Lab test
    - ☐ Observed
    - ☐ Assisted

    Brief summary:

    ____

    ____

Student Name: ______________________________

Technician Name: ______________________________

Notes

Student ______________________ Dates ____________ Site ____________ Preceptor ____________

Urinary Post-Clinical Reflection

Rotation Report

Overview

Instructions: Answer the following questions using complete sentences.

1. What were your responsibilities or duties this week?

2. What new knowledge or skill did you learn or observe this week?

3. What was the best thing that happened at your clinical site this week?

4. What was the most challenging thing that happened at your clinical site this week?

5. What problems or difficulties did you encounter or observe at your clinical site? How were they dealt with?

6. Was this week good, fair, or bad? Explain.

Observations

Instructions: List the observations you made for each of the following categories.

1. Technology observed:

2. Diagnostic procedures observed:

(Continued)

3. Therapeutic procedures observed:

____

____

4. Diseases or disorders observed:

____

____

5. Medical terminology or abbreviations encountered:

____

____

6. Other observations:

____

____

Supervisor Signature: ______________________________

Date: ______________________________

Rotation Journal

Instructions: Write a journal entry detailing your learning experience at the clinical rotation. Use the following topics to help write a complete journal entry.

Assessment of the Environment

- Personnel
- Services provided
- Equipment
- Technology utilized

Observation

- Health care providers
- Team skills
- Communication skills
- Safety procedures
- Therapeutic/diagnostic procedures

Knowledge

- New information learned
- Medical terminology
- Skills learned

Evaluation

- Personal experience
- Educational value
- Professional value

Journal Entry

Write a journal entry summarizing your clinical experience.

____

____

____

____

____

____